W9-CAV-480

NURSING PHOTOBOOK™

Managing I.V. Therapy

NURSING83 BOOKS™
INTERMED COMMUNICATIONS, INC.
SPRINGHOUSE, PENNSYLVANIA

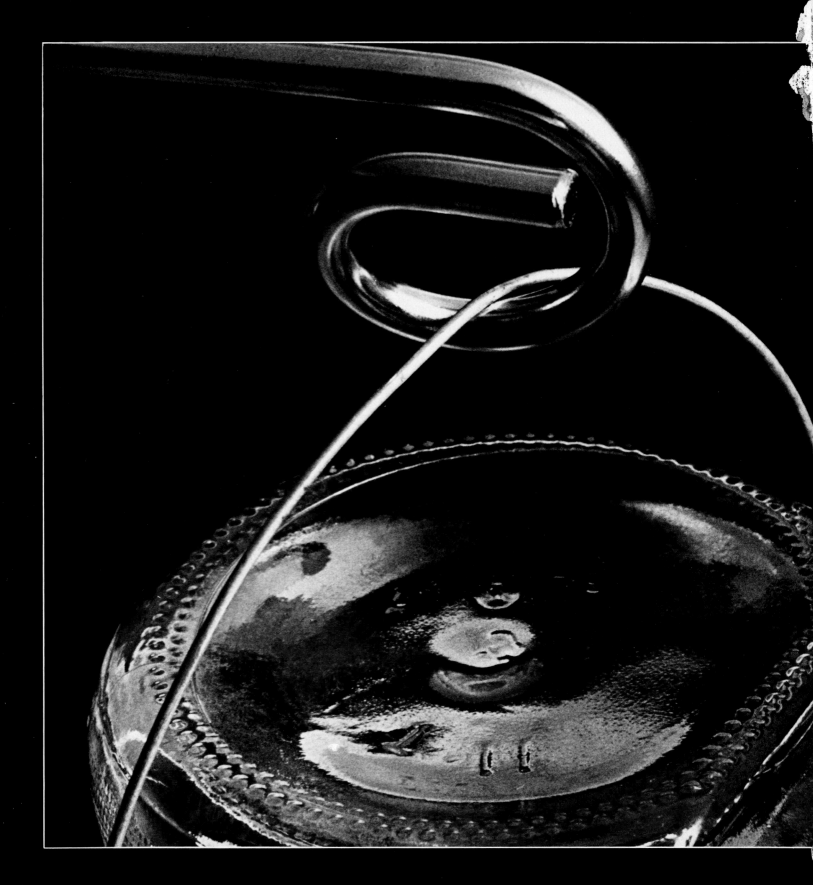

NURSING PHOTOBOOK

Managing
I.V. Therapy

NURSING83 BOOKS™

NURSING PHOTOBOOK™ SERIES
Providing Respiratory Care
Managing I.V. Therapy
Dealing with Emergencies
Giving Medications
Assessing Your Patients
Using Monitors
Providing Early Mobility
Giving Cardiac Care
Performing GI Procedures
Implementing Urologic Procedures
Controlling Infection
Ensuring Intensive Care
Coping with Neurologic Disorders
Caring for Surgical Patients
Working with Orthopedic Patients
Nursing Pediatric Patients
Helping Geriatric Patients
Attending Ob/Gyn Patients
Aiding Ambulatory Patients
Carrying Out Special Procedures

NURSING SKILLBOOK® SERIES
Reading EKGs Correctly
Dealing with Death and Dying
Managing Diabetics Properly
Assessing Vital Functions Accurately
Helping Cancer Patients Effectively
Giving Cardiovascular Drugs Safely
Giving Emergency Care Competently
Monitoring Fluid and Electrolytes Precisely
Documenting Patient Care Responsibly
Combatting Cardiovascular Diseases Skillfully
Coping with Neurologic Problems Proficiently
Using Crisis Intervention Wisely
Nursing Critically Ill Patients Confidently

NURSE'S REFERENCE LIBRARY®
Diseases
Diagnostics
Drugs
Assessment
Procedures

***Nursing83* DRUG HANDBOOK™**

NURSING PHOTOBOOK™ Series

PUBLISHER
Eugene W. Jackson

EDITORIAL DIRECTOR
Jean Robinson

CLINICAL DIRECTOR
Barbara McVan, RN

ART DIRECTOR
Lisa A. Gilde

**Intermed Communications
Book Division**

DIRECTOR
Timothy B. King

DIRECTOR, RESEARCH
Elizabeth O'Brien

DIRECTOR, PRODUCTION AND PURCHASING
Bacil Guiley

Staff for this volume

BOOK EDITOR
Richard Samuel West

CLINICAL EDITOR
Helene Ritting Nawrocki, RN

ASSOCIATE EDITOR
Katherine W. Carey

PHOTOGRAPHER
Paul A. Cohen

DESIGN DIRECTOR
Burton P. Pollack

DESIGNER
Linda Jovinelly Franklin

EDITORIAL/GRAPHIC COORDINATOR
Doreen K. Stowers

COPY EDITOR
Barbara Hodgson

EDITORIAL STAFF ASSISTANT
Evelyn M. James

ASSISTANT PHOTOGRAPHER
Thomas Staudenmayer

ART PRODUCTION MANAGER
Wilbur D. Davidson

ARTISTS
Lorraine Carbo   Robert Perry
Darcy Feralio   Sandra Simms
Diane Fox   Ron Yablon
Deborah Lugar

RESEARCHER AND INDEXER
Vonda Heller

TYPOGRAPHY MANAGER
David C. Kosten

TYPOGRAPHY ASSISTANTS
Diane Paluba
Thomas E. Roch

PRODUCTION MANAGER
Robert L. Dean, Jr.

PRODUCTION ASSISTANT
M. Eileen Hunsicker

ILLUSTRATORS
Jack Crane   John R. Murphy
Jean Gardner   Henry Rothman
Robert Jackson   Lynn Waldo
Cynthia Mason   Bud Yingling

SERIES GRAPHIC DESIGNER
John C. Isely

CONTRIBUTING PHOTOGRAPHERS
Robert Goldstein
Carroll H. Weiss

COVER PHOTO
Seymour Mednick

**Clinical consultants
for this volume**
Faye Cosentino, RN, BS
Director, Intravenous Therapy
Lawrence Hospital
Bronxville, New York

Lavenia Green Coleman, RN
Director, Intravenous Therapy
Temple University Health Sciences Center
Philadelphia, Pennsylvania

Home care aids and other specified pages in this book may be reproduced by office copier for distribution to patients. Written permission is required for any other use or to copy any other material in this book.

© 1983, 1979 by Intermed Communications, Inc., 1111 Bethlehem Pike, Springhouse, Pa. 19477. All rights reserved. Reproduction in whole or part by any means whatsoever without written permission of the publisher is prohibited by law. Printed in the United States of America.
PB-071282

Library of Congress Cataloging in Publication Data

Main entry under title:

Managing I.V. Therapy.

(Nursing Photobook)
Bibliography: p.
Includes index.
1. Intravenous therapy.   2. Nursing.
[DNLM: 1. Injections, Intravenous.   WB354 M266]
RM170.M36   615'.63   79-28050
ISBN 0-916730-18-2

Contents

Contributors

At the time of original publication, these contributors held the following positions.

Lavenia Green Coleman is director of I.V. therapy at Temple University Health Sciences Center, Philadelphia, Pennsylvania. A graduate of Kings County Hospital Center, School of Nursing, in Brooklyn, New York, she's a member of the National Intravenous Therapy Association (NITA). She is one of the advisors on this PHOTOBOOK.

Faye Cosentino, director of I.V. therapy at Lawrence Hospital, Bronxville, New York, earned a nursing diploma at Metropolitan Hospital School of Nursing and a BS degree at Mercy College, both in New York City. She belongs to NITA, the National Coordinating Committee for Large Volume Parenterals (NCCLVP), and the American Association of Blood Banks. She is one of the advisors on this PHOTOBOOK.

Nesbit Louise Jenkins supervises the I.V. therapy department at Lee Memorial Hospital in Fort Myers, Florida. She's a member of NITA and of the American Nurses' Association.

Susan Masoorli, a graduate of Misericordia Hospital in Philadelphia, is head nurse for the I.V. team at Pennsylvania Hospital in Philadelphia.

Rosemary Sadler Olson is nursing care coordinator of the intensive care unit at Metropolitan Medical Center in Minneapolis, Minnesota. She's a graduate of St. Barnabas School of Nursing, also in Minneapolis, and belongs to the American Association of Critical-Care Nurses.

Ira Spitzer, a pediatrician at Delaware Valley Medical Center, Bristol, Pennsylvania, and at Parkview Hospital, Philadelphia, Pennsylvania, earned a DO degree at the Philadelphia College of Osteopathic Medicine.

Penny Vail, a graduate of the Westchester School of Nursing, Valhalla, New York, supervises the I.V. therapy department at Florida Medical Center Hospital in Lauderdale Lakes. In 1978, she founded the Northeastern Chapter of NITA.

Introduction

You've been asking for it. A PHOTOBOOK illustrating the basics of intravenous therapy. Written and designed for you nurses who need practical, up-to-date help on the job. You already know how complex I.V. therapy can be, and you're probably a little scared of it. In addition, you may have difficulty with some of the procedures and questions about unfamiliar equipment.

For example, do you know how to work an infusion pump? How to calculate flow rates? Can you explain the difference between a piggyback and a secondary set, and do you know how to use each? Can you list the do's and don'ts of fat emulsion therapy? How do you deliver blood or blood components? How do you perform venipuncture safely and easily?

This PHOTOBOOK has the answers. In fact, you may come to think of it *as* the answer, because it *shows* you what to do at the same time it tells you. It guides you through each procedure step-by-step with clear, close-up photographs. And it presents the complex information you need to know in charts, illustrations, and diagrams.

Take a look at the contents page to see how much this PHOTOBOOK includes. You'll find all you need to know about I.V. equipment, including how to choose the correct needle or cannula. Performing venipuncture is illustrated in detail, with information on how to identify, correct, and prevent possible complications. Additionally, we'll show you the ins and outs of admixtures, the subtleties of using additive sets, and the special techniques of I.V. bolus.

You'll be led through the complicated steps of hyperalimentation and fat emulsion therapy, learning new ways to deal with old problems. We'll explore the detailed world of whole blood and its components. You'll get answers to often-asked questions about when to use which component and how to administer it. You'll also find out how to take a CVP reading, help perform a cutdown, and assist the doctor in inserting an umbilical line.

Keep an eye out for the logos and nursing tips which appear in color throughout this PHOTOBOOK. They clue you into important to-the-point information which will increase your knowledge and help you give better nursing care. Also, examine the children's coloring book feature in the back of the book. This patient teaching aid will delight your pediatric patients, and make your job of explaining I.V. therapy that much easier.

Everything you need is here in this illustrated guide to I.V. therapy. Study it. We think you'll agree it's invaluable.

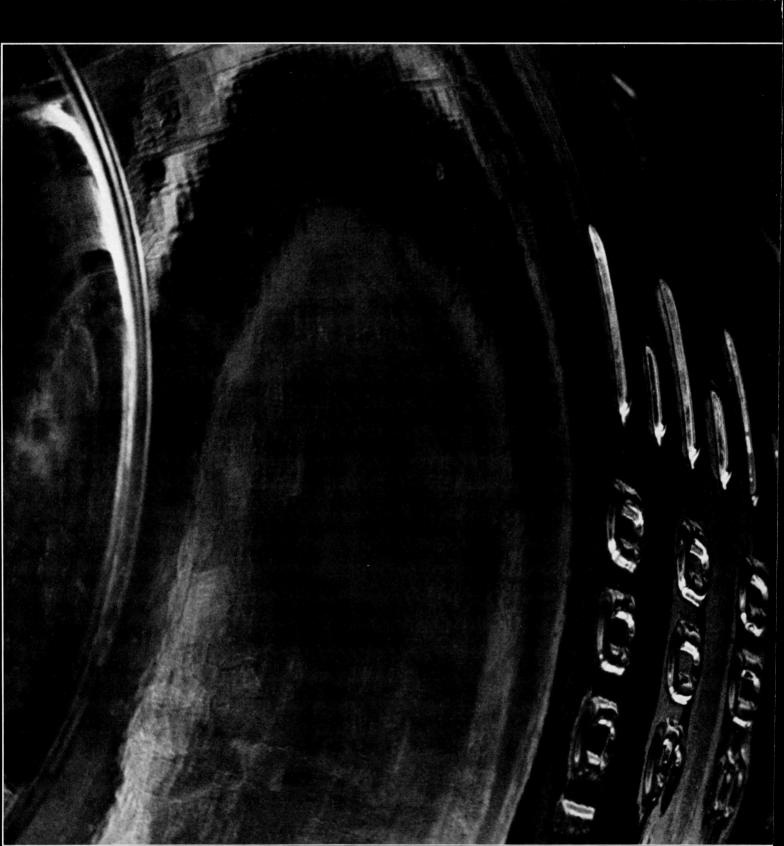

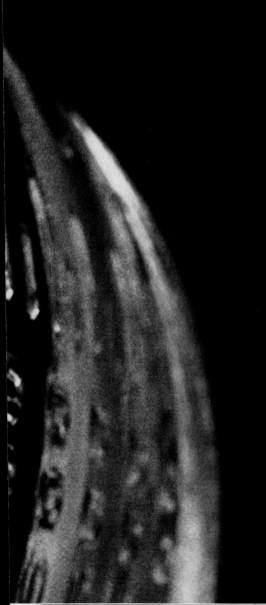

Preparing for I.V. Therapy

I.V. equipment

I.V. equipment

When we talk about I.V. therapy, we're discussing a wide variety of procedures, each used to treat a different health problem. Yet, all these procedures require the same basic equipment: antiseptic cleaning preparations, needles, syringes, tubing, bottles or bags, and dressings. When you learn how to use the equipment correctly, you learn the fundamentals of every procedure. Test your knowledge about I.V. therapy equipment. Do you know:
• Why an over-the-needle catheter's more prone to contamination than a winged-tip needle?
• When ethyl alcohol's used instead of iodine?
• Why a drip chamber must be half full before you prime the tubing?
• Why you should tap a filter during the priming process?

The answers to these questions, and others you probably have about I.V. therapy delivery systems, follow. Read this section before you read any other.

How I.V. contaminants are introduced

Before use

In infusion fluids or additives

Through punctures in plastic containers or cracks in glass bottles

Through vacuum-sealed bottle

In administration components

In attachments to primary and secondary ports

In disinfectants, prepping ointments, dressing materials

During use

In additives

During container changes

Through air filter

During tubing changes

During injections, irrigations, etc.

During CVP measurements

Through stopcock or other connections

During insertion and manipulation of cannula or needle

At insertion site

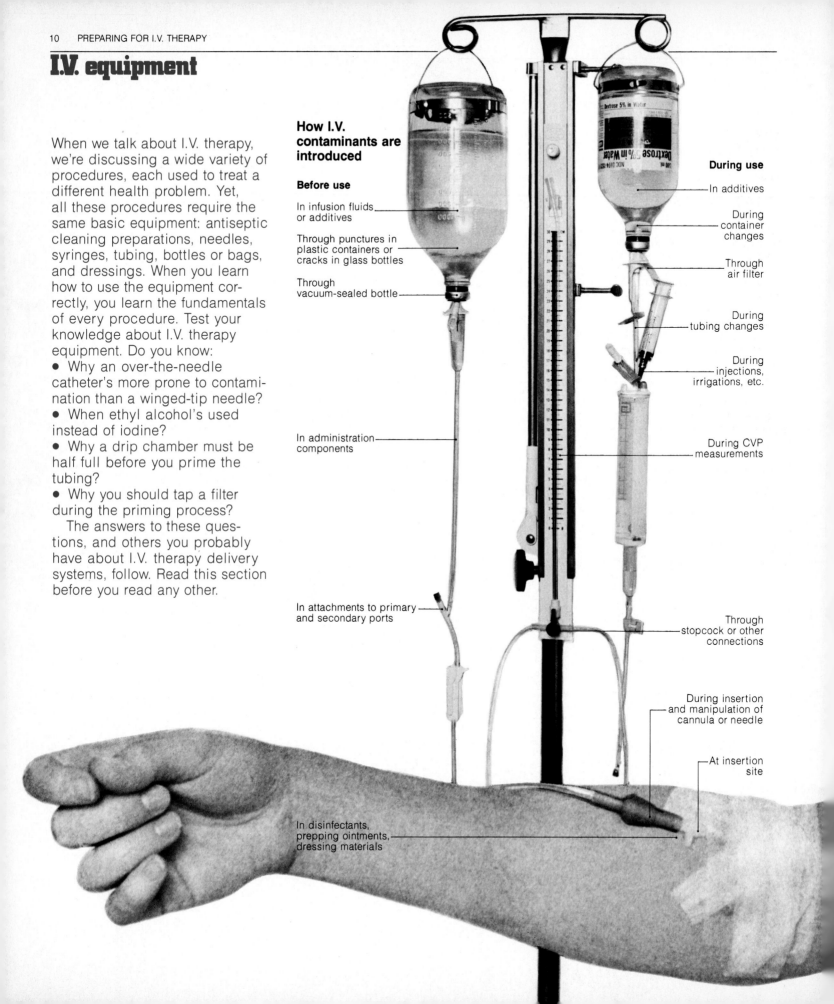

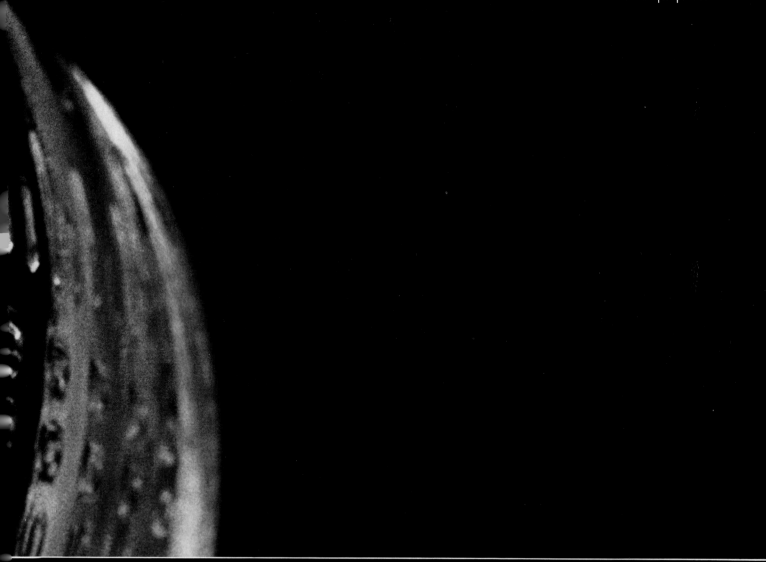

Preparing for
I.V. Therapy

I.V. equipment

I.V. equipment

When we talk about I.V. therapy, we're discussing a wide variety of procedures, each used to treat a different health problem. Yet, all these procedures require the same basic equipment: antiseptic cleaning preparations, needles, syringes, tubing, bottles or bags, and dressings. When you learn how to use the equipment correctly, you learn the fundamentals of every procedure. Test your knowledge about I.V. therapy equipment. Do you know:

• Why an over-the-needle catheter's more prone to contamination than a winged-tip needle?

• When ethyl alcohol's used instead of iodine?

• Why a drip chamber must be half full before you prime the tubing?

• Why you should tap a filter during the priming process?

The answers to these questions, and others you probably have about I.V. therapy delivery systems, follow. Read this section before you read any other.

How I.V. contaminants are introduced

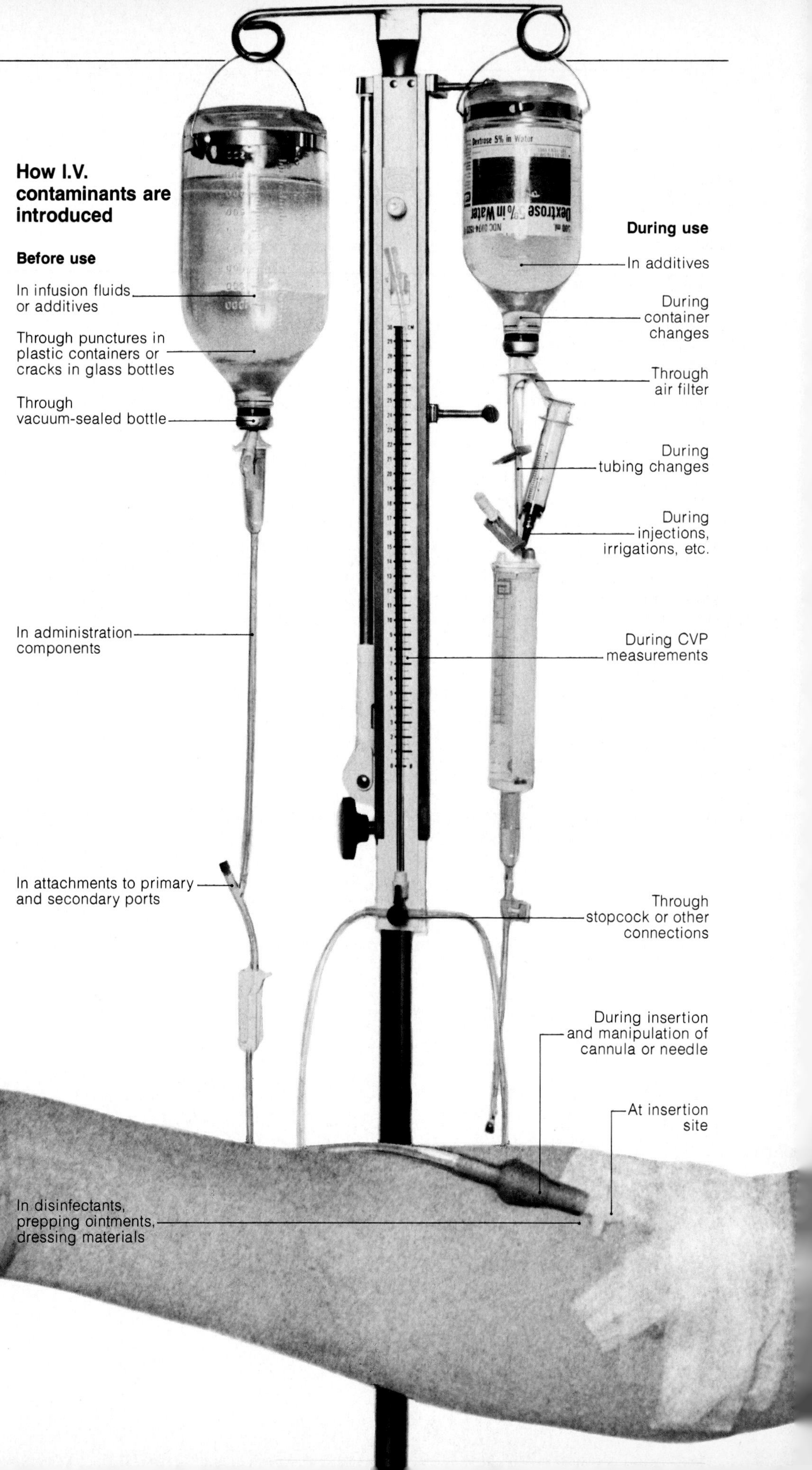

Before use

In infusion fluids or additives

Through punctures in plastic containers or cracks in glass bottles

Through vacuum-sealed bottle

In administration components

In attachments to primary and secondary ports

In disinfectants, prepping ointments, dressing materials

During use

In additives

During container changes

Through air filter

During tubing changes

During injections, irrigations, etc.

During CVP measurements

Through stopcock or other connections

During insertion and manipulation of cannula or needle

At insertion site

Questions to ask yourself when you inspect containers and solutions

Every aspect of I.V. therapy has potential troublespots. You can prevent or minimize these hazards by carefully inspecting the container and the solution. Never neglect these important steps.

1 To begin, examine the label and ask yourself:
• Is this the correct amount? Check the volume with the doctor's written order.
• Is this the correct solution? Match the label with the doctor's written order.
• Is the solution still fresh? Check the expiration date.

2 Next, examine the container and ask yourself: Is the glass intact? Does the bag have any dimples or puncture marks? To find out, hold the container up to the light and rotate it slowly. Cracks and chips in glass will reflect the light. Punctures in plastic will leak if you gently squeeze the bag.

You can safely ignore scratches on the container's surface, but don't dismiss any irregularities unless you're sure the solution's unaffected. Remember: Hairline cracks may not leak, but they can permit bacteria to infiltrate the solution.

Examine the solution and ask yourself: Is it clear? Hold it up to the light and slowly rotate it. If you see foreign matter or cloudiness, discard the container.

3 Examine the cap over the spike port on a bottle and over the additive port on a bag and ask yourself: Is the seal intact and secure? Don't use the container if it looks like it's been tampered with. (If the hospital pharmacy has added medication to the solution, they'll reseal the container with a sterile additive cap.)

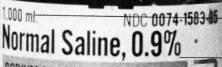

1,000 ml.   NDC 0074-1583-05
Normal Saline, 0.9%
SODIUM CHLORIDE INJECTION, U.S.P.

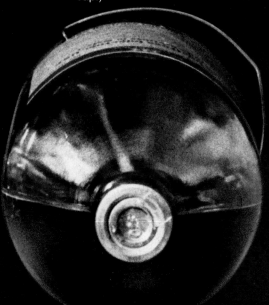

I.V. equipment

Selecting the correct line

You're about to establish an I.V. line. Which type should you choose? That depends on your needs. Each feature available on an I.V. line serves a special purpose. Check out the following. Then, decide what's best for your patient.

Microdrip   Macrodrip

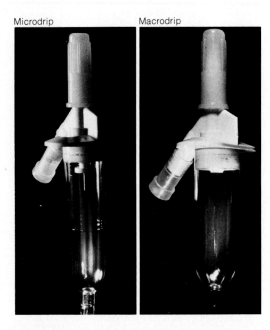

Drip systems

If you're delivering a small amount of solution or want to keep a vein open, a microdrip system (shown on the left) will serve you best. Why not use a macrodrip system for such cases? The reason is simple. With a macrodrip, you'll risk clotting the drip system because so much time will elapse between drops. Instead, use the macrodrip (shown on the right) when you want to deliver solutions in large quantities or at fast rates. For more detailed information about drip systems, see page 17.

Vented   Nonvented

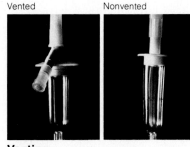

Venting

If you're using a standard bottle, you'll need vented tubing, as we show on the left. The vent will permit air to enter the vacuum in the bottle and displace the solution as it flows out. Select nonvented tubing if you're using a bag, because the bag will compress as the solution flows out. You also use it with a vented bottle, because the bottle has a built-in air vent.

Venting

Drip system

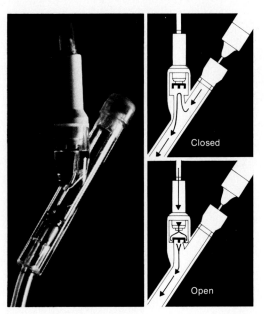

Closed

Open

Piggyback port

If you plan to administer medication intermittently during I.V. therapy, you'll need a line with a piggyback port, as shown here. We'll talk about piggyback lines later in the book, starting on page 71. Right now we're focusing on the port alone. The port features a backcheck valve, which automatically stops the I.V. solution from flowing and allows the piggyback solution to run, as shown in the drawing on the top right. Then, when the piggyback bottle empties, the backcheck valve starts the I.V. solution again, as shown in the bottom right drawing.

Piggyback port

Clamp

Secondary port

Filter

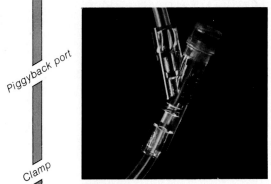

Secondary port

You'll use a secondary port when you want to run primary and secondary solutions. You can run each line individually, or you can run them simultaneously. For information on the sets that hook into the secondary port, see pages 71 and 72.

400

Clamp

Fluid chamber

Clamp

Secondary port

Filter

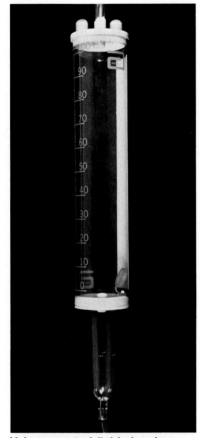

Volume-control fluid chamber (with attached drip chamber)
You'll use a line equipped with a volume-control fluid chamber (also known as a Soluset® or Buretrol® set) when you want to deliver small doses of medication or fluid over an extended period of time. You'll use the fluid chamber to measure the dose. Then, to ensure an accurate delivery, the medication passes through the drip chamber. A line with a fluid chamber won't have a piggyback port. For more details on volume-control fluid chambers, see page 79.

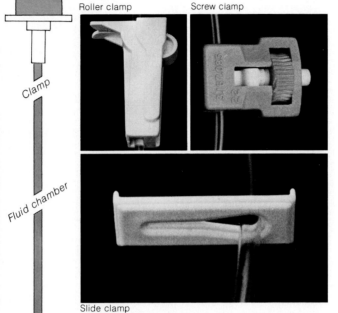

Roller clamp   Screw clamp

Slide clamp

Clamps
Every primary line's equipped with one or more clamps to regulate flow. Here are three different types. The top two can increase or decrease the flow. The third type simply stops or starts it.

The one on the top left is the roller clamp. To work it, use your thumb to move the roller up (opening the line) or down (closing the line). Top right is the screw clamp. Work it by turning it clockwise to close the line and counterclockwise to open the line. The lower photo shows the slide clamp, which will stop the flow when you slide the tube into the narrow end and start the flow again when you slide the tube into the wide end. This clamp should be used in combination with other clamps.

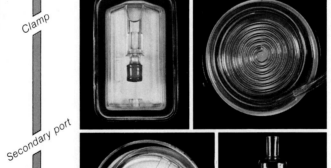
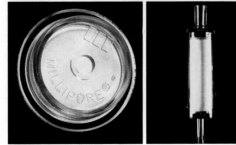

ACF filter   Continue-flo filter

Millipore filter   IVEX 2 filter

Filters
Filters help minimize the risk of contamination. As you can see in the photos at the left, they come in several sizes and shapes, but all work to reduce particulate matter in the solution you're delivering. Some filters come built into the line. Others must be attached. Read the manufacturer's instructions to make sure the filter you use is not finer than the solution you're passing through it. If it is, it'll clog. To learn how filters work and when to use them, see pages 20 and 21.

I.V. equipment

Spiking and priming

1 *Before you perform veni-puncture on a patient, you must spike the container and run I.V. fluid through the tubing to expel all the air. This simple but important process is called priming.*

Begin by washing your hands thoroughly. Then, gather your equipment: a bottle or bag of the prescribed I.V. solution, the proper tubing, and an I.V. pole.

2 Now, slide the flow clamp along the tubing until it's directly under the drip chamber. Then, close the clamp.

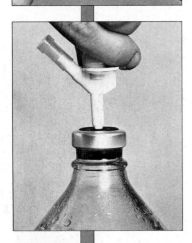

3 Get ready to spike the container. Suppose you're using a bottle with a rubber stopper, like the one in this photo. Remove the protective metal cap, and swab the stopper with alcohol. Place the bottle on a stable surface, and steady it by holding the stopper between your finger and thumb. Then, remove the plastic cover from the spike, and push the spike firmly into the rubber stopper. To make sure the spike's in far enough, watch for it in the bottle neck.

4 Some bottles, like this one, have an indwelling vent and a latex diaphragm. In this case, you'd use nonvented tubing. Before spiking, remove both the protective metal cap and the diaphragm. Listen for a hiss of inrushing air, indicating a vacuum. (If you don't hear a hiss, discard the bottle. No vacuum means the bottle's been contaminated.)

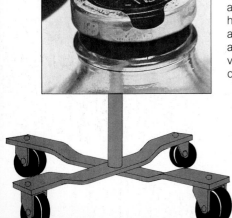

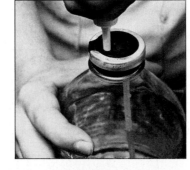

5 Is the bottle O.K.? Then continue. Look for the two holes under the diaphragm. Insert the spike into the larger hole *without* an air vent.

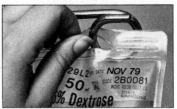

6 Spiking a bag's a little different. The type pictured in this photo should be hung before spiking. Otherwise, the pressure from your hand as you grasp the port and bag may expel the air needed to read the fluid level accurately.

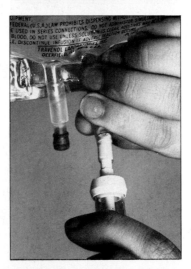

7 Now, steady the port with one hand, and remove its protective cap by pulling smoothly to the *right*. Pulling to the left may rip the cap's tab in two. When you've done this, insert a nonvented spike into the port with one quick, smooth motion. If you hesitate, fluid may escape before you've completed the insertion.

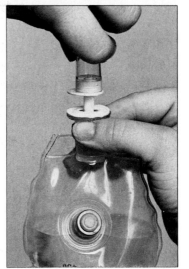

8 Here's another kind of bag. To remove it's protective cap, just pull the tab. Because this bag has a firm, easy-to-grip port with a large lip guarding against touch contamination, you can spike it before hanging. Grasp it firmly by the port, but don't squeeze the bag or you'll force out the air. Then, insert the spike, and hang the bag so the injection port's facing away from the I.V. pole.

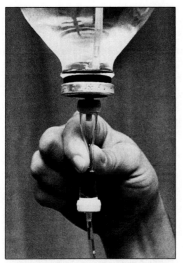

9 Now your container's spiked and hanging. Gently squeeze the drip chamber until it's half full. If you prime the tubing without doing this first, air bubbles may form in the drip chamber and travel down the tubing.

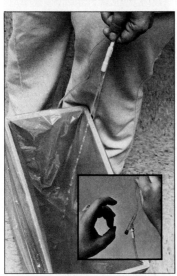

10 Here's how to prime the tubing. First, hold the end of it over a sink, wastebasket, or paper cup. Remove the protective cap. (Keep the cap from becoming contaminated, because you'll be using it again. Either set it down carefully with the open end up, or hold it, taking care not to touch the inside.)

Now, unclamp the tubing. Let the fluid run, as shown in this photo, until it fills the tubing and all air bubbles have been expelled. If you see small bubbles near the top of the tubing or in the drip chamber, lightly tap the area until the bubbles rise into the container.
[Inset] If your tubing has a backcheck valve on it, invert the valve as you prime. Gently tap the valve with your finger to remove air bubbles.

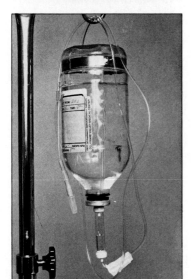

11 Clamp off the tubing, and replace the protective cap. Loop the tubing over the I.V. pole, so it's out of the way while you perform venipuncture. (Some flow clamps have a V-shaped hook to hold the tubing.)

Remember: Always label the container and tubing with date and time of insertion, and type of solution. We'll discuss exactly how to do this on page 43.

Hanging the I.V. container: Some options

Your best bet for hanging an I.V. container is a standard I.V. pole, because it's safe and can easily be adjusted to the correct height. However, in a pinch, use your imagination. For example, if the patient's bed has a curtain around it, temporarily hang the bottle or bag on one of the hooks. Or use the hook on the back of a bathroom door (if it's placed high enough) when an ambulatory patient doesn't want to wheel his pole into the bathroom. A curtain hook rigged up on a window blind works too. Just remember these important restrictions when you're improvising temporary hangers:
● Make sure the hook's secure.
● Keep the container about 3' (1 m) above the insertion site at all times.

Calculating flow rates

To calculate the right flow rate for your patient, answer these questions:
● How much solution did the doctor order?
● How much time is allowed for delivery?
Take the amount of solution to be administered and divide it by the delivery time; for example,

$$\frac{1000 \text{ ml}}{8 \text{ hours}} = 125 \text{ ml per hour.}$$

Now, decide which type of drip system you're using. If you're delivering a lot of fluid in a short time, use a macrodrip system. The macrodrip, depending on the manufacturer, takes 10, 15, or 20 drops to deliver 1 ml. If you're delivering a small amount of fluid over a long time, use a microdrip system. The microdrip takes 60 drops to deliver 1 ml.
Insert your answers into this formula:

$$\frac{\text{drops per ml}}{60 \text{ minutes per hour}} \times \frac{\text{amount of fluid per hour}}{1} = \frac{\text{drops}}{\text{per minute}}$$

If you're using a macrodrip system, your equation will look like one of these:

$$\frac{10}{60} \times \frac{125}{1} = \frac{125}{6} = 21 \text{ drops per minute}$$

$$\frac{15}{60} \times \frac{125}{1} = \frac{125}{4} = 31 \text{ drops per minute}$$

$$\frac{20}{60} \times \frac{125}{1} = \frac{125}{3} = 41 \text{ drops per minute}$$

If you're using a microdrip system, your equation will look like this:

$$\frac{60}{60} \times \frac{125}{1} = 125 \text{ drops per minute}$$

After you've determined the rate, setting the flow is easy. When you've established your I.V. line, slowly open the clamp to start fluid dripping into the drip chamber. Hold your watch close to the chamber, and time the drips for 1 minute. Open or close the clamp, as needed, to adjust the drip rate. *Remember:* Anytime the clamp slips, for whatever reason, or the patient makes a sudden move, the drip rate may be affected. Check it periodically, using the method described above. Remind the patient and his family not to tamper with the clamp.

I.V. equipment

Getting acquainted with needles and cannulas

Take a good look at these needles and cannulas. They're among your most important I.V. tools. The outside diameter of the needle shaft is called a gauge. The larger the gauge number, the smaller the diameter of the shaft. The inside diameter of the shaft is called the lumen. Today, most needles (and some catheters) are coated with silicone, which makes insertion smoother and clotting less likely. They have short, sharp bevels to minimize trauma and pain during insertion. In addition, they're disposable.

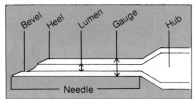

On the top right is a winged-tip, or butterfly, needle. It comes in lengths of ½" to 1¼". Diameters range from 25G to 17G. The wings attached to the shaft are made of rubber or plastic, and the flexible tubing extending behind them may be from 3" to 12" long.

The over-the-needle catheter (ONC) consists of a needle with a catheter fitted around it, as the photo in the center shows. The catheter is from 1¼" to 5½" long and from 12G to 22G in diameter. The point of the needle extends beyond the tip of the catheter. After venipuncture, you'll withdraw and discard the needle, leaving just the catheter in the vein. *Note:* For clarity, we'll call any needle/catheter set a *cannula*.

On the bottom right is an inside-the-needle catheter (INC). The cannula consists of a catheter between 14G and 19G in diameter lying inside a needle. The needle may be from 1½" to 2" long, and the catheter from 8" to 36" long. The clear plastic sleeve over the catheter protects it from touch contamination during insertion. When the catheter's in place, you'll withdraw the needle and secure it outside the skin in a protective bevel cover. Since the catheter is radiopaque, you can confirm proper placement with an X-ray.

Nurses' guide to needles and catheters

Winged-tip

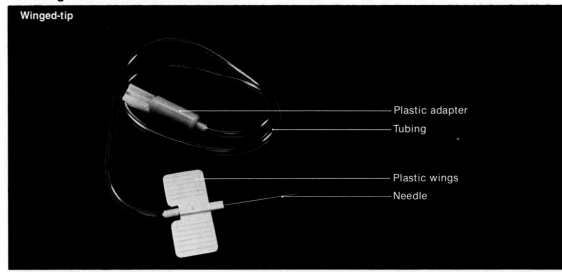

Over-the-needle catheter
(ONC)

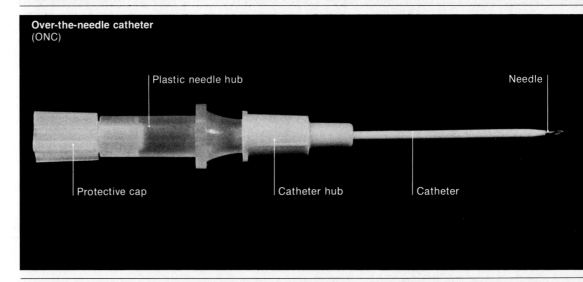

Inside-the-needle catheter
(INC)

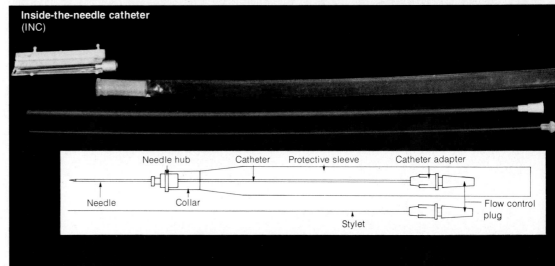

Used for	Advantages	Disadvantages
• Infants and children • The elderly and other adults with small veins • Adults receiving short-term therapy	• Simple, easy to use • Relatively painless insertion • The wings reduce the risk of touch contamination	• Less stable than indwelling catheters • Not suitable for delivery of highly viscous liquids or for long-term therapy • Needle point may damage vein during therapy, causing infiltration
• Long-term therapy • Delivery of viscous liquids, like blood or hyperalimentation fluid • Arterial monitoring	• Less likely to damage the vein during therapy than a winged-tip needle • Needle can be completely removed after insertion, greatly reducing the risk of catheter embolus. • No blood leakage, since the puncture made by the needle's just the right size for the catheter • Stable; allows greater patient mobility than the winged-tip needle.	• More likely to damage the vein during insertion than a winged-tip needle • Prone to touch contamination • The plastic catheter's more likely to support infection and trigger phlebitis than a metal needle. • Catheter embolus may result if the catheter's withdrawn over the needle.
• Long-term therapy • Delivery of viscous liquids • Delivery of drugs to central veins • Central venous pressure monitoring	• Permits insertion of catheter into superior vena cava or heart by peripheral route • Less likely to damage the vein than a winged-tip needle • Stable • Plastic sleeve reduces the risk of touch contamination.	• Needle remains secured outside the skin, risking catheter embolus if it's not well secured with sutures and/or tape. • Catheter embolus is likely if catheter's withdrawn through the needle. • Plastic catheter may support infection or trigger phlebitis. • Some bleeding may occur after venipuncture when needle's withdrawn.

Choosing the correct needle and catheter

Needles and catheters come in a bewildering array of lengths and diameters. Choosing what's best for your patient isn't always easy, but as a rule, the smaller the size, the better. A small needle and catheter cause less trauma to the vein. They also allow greater blood flow around the tip, reducing the risk of clotting.

Using a catheter that's too big for the vein invites complications. However, if a large-sized catheter *must* be used for viscous fluids like blood, choose a larger vein to accommodate it.

Before deciding which needle and catheter to use, consider the age, size, and condition of your patient. Keep these guidelines in mind:
• For most routine venipunctures on adults, use small (20G to 22G) needles and catheters.
• For venipunctures on infants and children, use a short (½") winged-tip needle.
• Because arteries lie deeper in the tissues than veins, use a longer needle (1½" to 2") for arterial punctures.

Some procedures may require specific equipment. For example, the doctor will probably choose an inside-the-needle catheter (INC) with a 12" catheter to perform a subclavian insertion. However, for a small patient, an 8" catheter will probably be long enough. But if the subclavian's being entered by a peripheral route, most adults will need a 24" catheter.

What if the doctor decides to do a cutdown? He'll probably insert a cutdown catheter directly into the incision site. A cutdown catheter's from 8" to 12" in length and 12G to 22G in diameter, depending on the vein chosen for the cutdown. Like most intravenous catheters, it's radiopaque so you can locate it easily if a catheter embolus occurs.

PRECAUTIONS

Inspecting a needle or catheter

Do you always assume that new equipment is flawless? Don't be too sure! Defects can occur. And if you don't spot them, your patient's health may suffer.

Whenever you unpack a needle or cannula, look at it closely. You may find one of these defects:
• Barbs or roughness on the needle bevel
• Bumps or frayed edges on the catheter tip
• Errors in labeling or packaging.

Important: Avoid contaminating the equipment with your hands when you unpack and examine it. Open packages according to the manufacturer's instructions—*not* by punching the needle or cannula through the wrapping. Check for defects by sight only.

I.V. equipment

Why use a filter?

Have you ever thought, "If my line's sterile and the solution I'm infusing has been prepared under sterile conditions, why do I also need a filter?" The answer is simple. No matter how many precautions you've taken beforehand, contamination's always a possibility. Here's a list of particulate matter that could be in the solution you're ready to administer:

• Dissolved impurities in water, like detergents, proteins, and polysaccharides

• Inorganic impurities in water, like salt from soil, rocks, pipes, and tanks

• Microorganisms, which, if alive, will multiply in the bloodstream or, if dead, will enter the tissue and cause a sterile abscess

• Particles of metal, lint, asbestos, rubber, cotton, dust, or glass

• Undissolved drug powders or crystals

• Precipitates from incompatible admixtures.

Considering these possibilities, you can see why a filter's so important. Use a filter whenever:

• an additive has been combined with the solution

• the injection port on the tubing will be used

• the patient's especially susceptible to infusion phlebitis or infection

• the infusion will be given centrally.

Filter membranes come in several sizes, ranging from 5 microns (the largest) to 0.22 micron (the smallest). They allow liquids but not particles to pass through them. The finer the membrane, the more fully it'll filter the liquid. Here's how size relates to the filter's function:

• 5 to 1 micron filters remove most particulate matter, but not most fungi or bacteria

• 0.45 micron filters remove fungi and most bacteria

• 0.22 micron filters remove virtually all fungi and bacteria but reduce flow rate, which, of course, is crucial when you need extremely rapid administration.

Anatomy of a filter

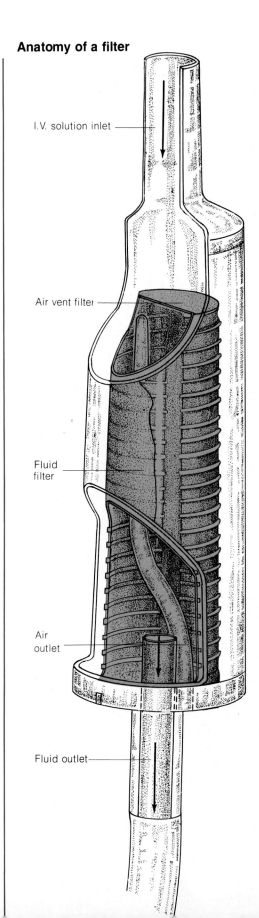

I.V. solution inlet

Air vent filter

Fluid filter

Air outlet

Fluid outlet

How to add and prime a filter

1 *Suppose the doctor tells you to add a filter to an I.V. administration set. Will you know how? This photostory will show you.*

As you begin, remember that you must always use aseptic technique to connect one part of a delivery system to another. (For details on this, see page 11.) Then, once you've minimized the risk of contamination, proceed as follows. First, remove the caps from the administration set and the filter. Fit the tubing's male adapter into the filter's female connector. Twist it firmly to make a snug connection.

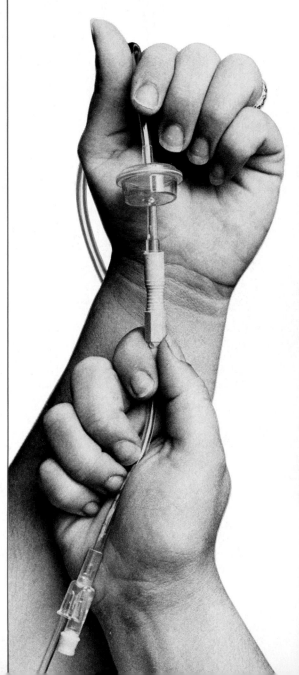

2 Next, hold the filter so the male-female joint is pointed down, as shown in this photo. Then, open all the clamps on the line to prime the tubing and the filter.

As the solution runs, tap the filter, working from the bottom up. This'll dislodge any air bubbles that may be trapped in the membrane. When that's completed, close the roller clamp. Now you're ready to start venipuncture.

3 If the filter's built into the line, like the one shown in this photo, prime it in the same way. But when you're ready to infuse the solution, follow the manufacturer's recommendations on the filter's position. Most filters should be upright, but some should stay inverted during use.

Needle filters: How they work

Sometimes you'll need to filter medication as you draw it into the syringe. In those cases, you can use a filter needle (a needle with a built-in filter). But what if one's not handy? Then, *make* a filter needle by following these simple steps:

• Pull back the tabs on the add-a-filter and the needle packages, following the manufacturer's directions.

• Hold the add-a-filter in the center, and remove the protective cap.

• Fit the filter into the needle hub and place the filter and needle unit on a syringe.

Important: Discard the filter needle, and replace it with a regular needle after you've drawn the medication.

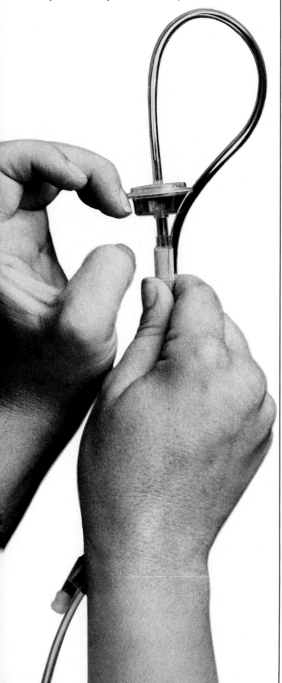

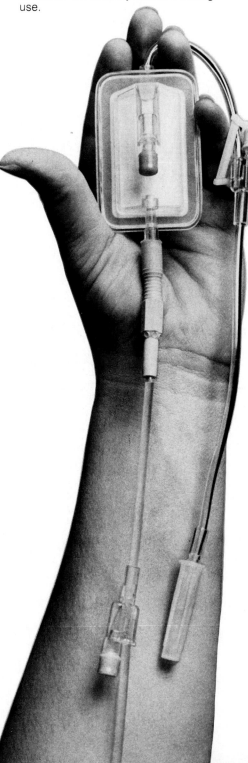

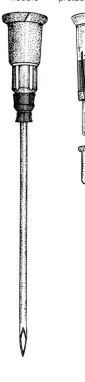

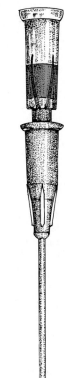

Filter needle

Add-a-filter with protective cap

Needle with add-a-filter

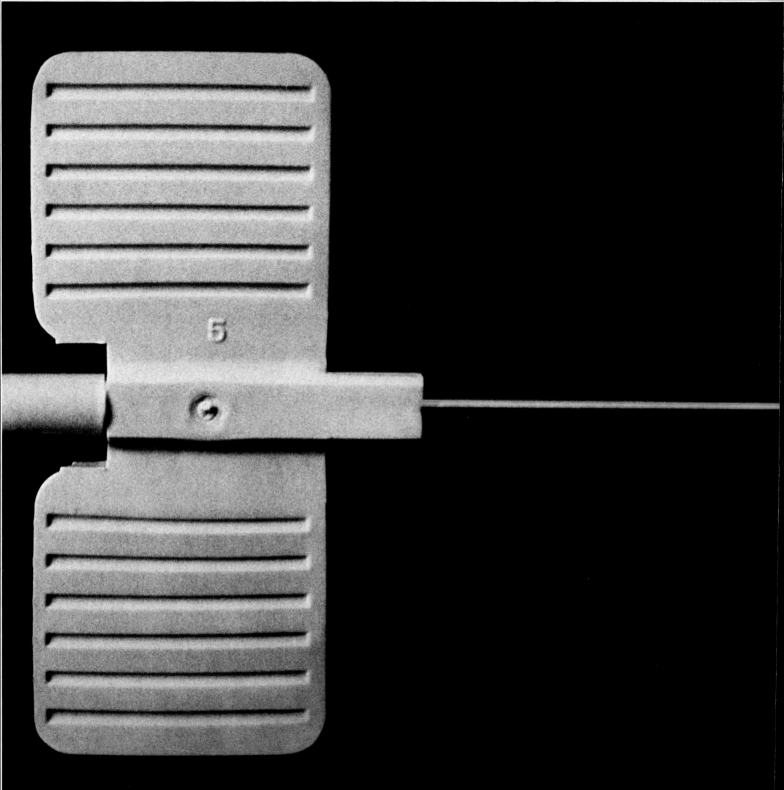

Performing Basic I.V. Procedures

Venipuncture

"I wish I didn't have to do venipunctures. I'm so afraid I'll miss the patient's vein and hurt him unnecessarily." Have you ever said anything like this? Venipuncture—the procedure for entering a vein with a needle or a catheter—takes some practice, but it's easier to master than you may think.

Maybe you've never seen step-by-step demonstrations of venipuncture techniques or understood the reasoning behind them. If you haven't, you'll find the following pages invaluable. But even if you're experienced at I.V. therapy, you'll find lots of tips that'll help you do your job even better.

Here are a few of the procedures and skills we'll cover:
● How to select and dilate a vein
● How to insert a needle and cannula
● How to care for both patient and equipment during I.V. therapy
● How to recognize problems and deal with them.

Venipuncture's basic to I.V. therapy. By understanding it thoroughly, you'll find it easier to perform procedures with confidence.

INDICATIONS/CONTRAINDICATIONS

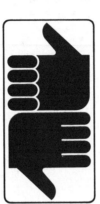

Knowing when to use venipuncture

Venipuncture's indicated when you must:
● Maintain or correct fluid and electrolyte balance.
● Administer continuous or intermittent medication.
● Administer blood or blood components.
● Administer a bolus preparation.
● Obtain blood samples for lab tests.
● Monitor CVP.
● Administer an intravenous anesthetic.
● Nourish a patient who can't eat normally.
● Keep a vein open in case of emergency.
● Perform a phlebotomy.

Venipuncture's contraindicated when:
● Oral medication can be given effectively.
● Intramuscular medication can be given effectively and comfortably. (However, a thin patient, or one who needs frequent injections, probably will be happier with an I.V. line.)
● The patient's sensitive or allergic to I.V. medication or equipment.
● The patient has a coagulation disorder (unless, of course, the I.V.'s needed to treat the condition).
● The patient's lucid and refuses I.V. treatment.

PATIENT PREPARATION

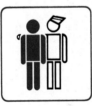

Preparing the patient for venipuncture

Even if venipuncture's routine for you, your patient may see it as a new experience. In addition, he may be apprehensive about the procedure and concerned that his condition's worsened. And if he's a child, his fears may be completely unrealistic. For example, he may think he's about to be poisoned, or that the needle will never be removed. So, help your patient relax. Take the mystery out of venipuncture by anticipating and answering all his questions.

Always begin by double-checking the patient's identity. Ask him his name and check his wristband. Then, ask if he's ever had an I.V. before. Be supportive if he's fearful; consider having another nurse hold his hand while you work.

Explain to him:
● why he needs I.V. therapy
● how venipuncture's done
● how much discomfort he'll feel
● how therapy will limit his activities
● how he can help keep the infusion flowing properly. For example, tell him *not* to manipulate the needle or flow clamp, and to call a nurse if he notices a change in the flow rate.

If the patient's agitated, try to postpone the procedure until he's calmer. Since tension makes the veins constrict, his cooperation is important. If he's still anxious despite your efforts to quiet him, a mild sedative may help. Occasionally, the doctor may have to order restraints; for example, when a patient's combative. (For details on how to apply restraints, see page 45.)

When your patient's as calm as possible, put him in a supine position, with his head slightly elevated. Make sure the room's quiet and well lighted. This will help your patient relax and will increase your ability to concentrate.

Important: If, for some reason, you aren't successful with venipuncture after two attempts, ask someone who's more experienced to take over.

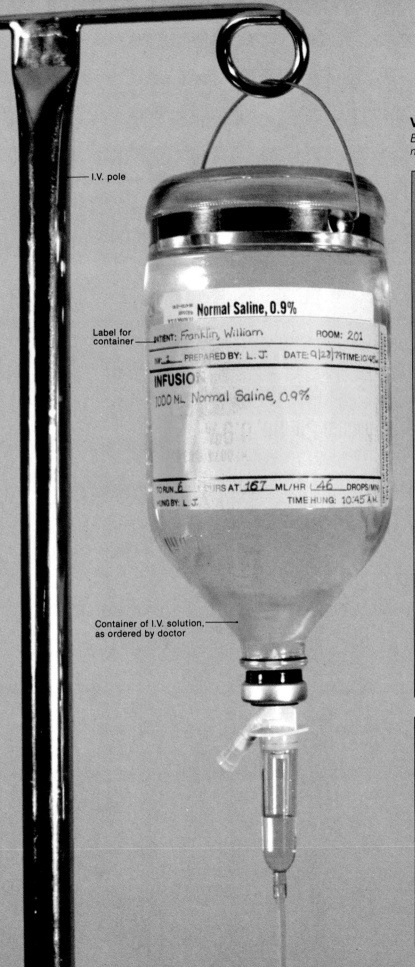

I.V. pole

Label for
container

Container of I.V. solution,
as ordered by doctor

Normal Saline, 0.9%

PATIENT: Franklin, William   ROOM: 201

IV. 1   PREPARED BY: L. J.   DATE: 9|23|79 TIME: 10:45

INFUSION
1000 ML Normal Saline, 0.9%

TO RUN 6 HOURS AT 167 ML/HR 46 DROPS/MIN

HUNG BY: L. J.   TIME HUNG: 10:45 A.M.

Venipuncture: Gathering your equipment

Before you begin venipuncture, assemble all the equipment you'll need, and remember to thoroughly wash your hands.

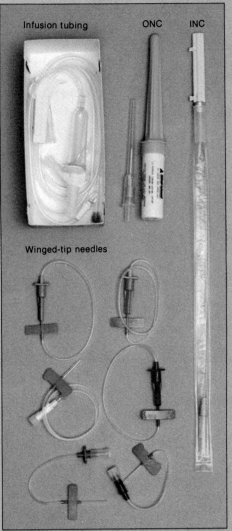

Infusion tubing   ONC   INC

Winged-tip needles

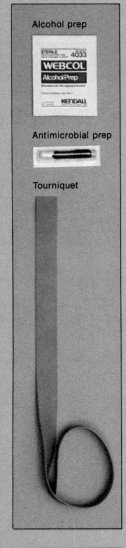

Alcohol prep

STERILE 4033
WEBCOL
Alcohol Prep

Antimicrobial prep

Tourniquet

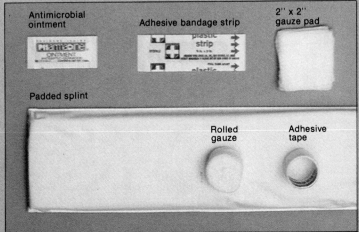

Antimicrobial
ointment   Adhesive bandage strip   2" x 2"
gauze pad

plastic
strip

plastic

Padded splint

Rolled
gauze   Adhesive
tape

Venipuncture

Nurses' guide to the anatomy of venipuncture sites

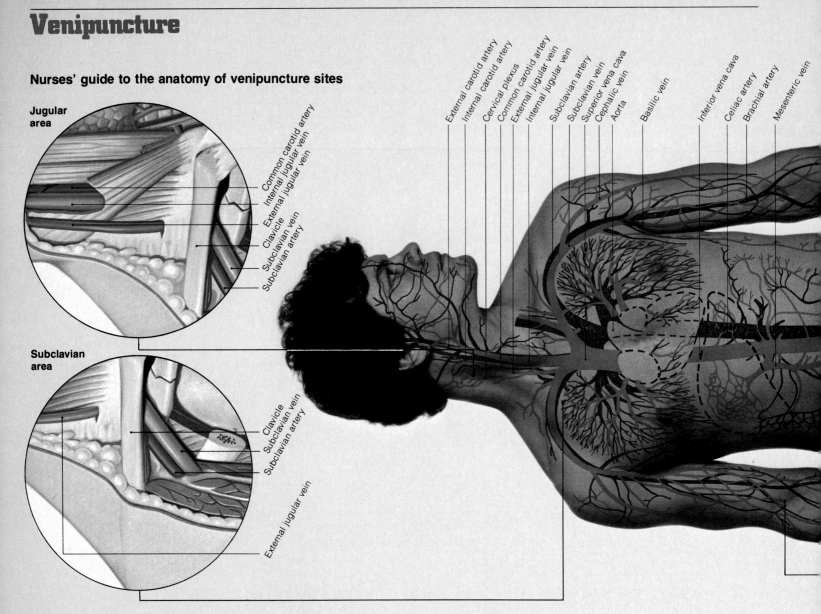

Jugular area

Common carotid artery
Internal jugular vein
External jugular vein
Clavicle
Subclavian vein
Subclavian artery

Subclavian area

Clavicle
Subclavian artery
Subclavian vein
External jugular vein

External carotid artery
Internal carotid artery
Cervical plexus
Common carotid artery
External jugular vein
Internal jugular vein
Subclavian artery
Subclavian vein
Superior vena cava
Cephalic vein
Aorta
Basilic vein
Inferior vena cava
Celiac artery
Brachial artery
Mesenteric vein

Andrew Olson's a 66-year-old man suffering from a persistent case of influenza. Because he's dehydrated, his doctor orders I.V. therapy to replace lost body fluids. Your job is to perform the venipuncture. Do you know which site is best for Mr. Olson?

Consider these guidelines. For an adult, the best venipuncture sites, in order of preference, are the lower arm and hand, the upper arm, and the antecubital fossa. (The lower extremities are undesirable because they're prone to thrombophlebitis and embolism.) Whenever possible, use the distal end of the vein. But don't make a choice without considering these factors as well:

• *How long will I.V. therapy last?* For short-term therapy, use the left arm or hand if your patient's right-handed; his right arm or hand if he's left-handed. For long-term therapy, alternate arms and avoid sites over joints.

• *What kind of I.V. solution's been ordered?* Infusions that are highly acidic, alkaline, or hypertonic can irritate a small peripheral vein; a larger vein will dilute the infusion better. Rapid infusions also require larger veins. (If no large peripheral veins are available, the doctor may decide to use a central vein. We'll discuss this in detail, beginning on page 90.)

• *What size needle or cannula are you using?* If the solution's highly viscous, you'll need one with a large bore. Choose a vein

that's big enough to accommodate it.

• *Is the vein full, soft, and unobstructed?* Palpate to find a vein that's not crooked, hardened, scarred, or inflamed. If you must use a lower extremity, carefully check for varicosity *above* the venipuncture site. 🕮 *Nursing tip:* When you must use a varicose vein, help prevent problems by elevating the limb during the infusion.

But what if the patient's veins are neither visible nor palpable? You may find a fiberoptic illuminator helpful. To use it, turn off the room lights, and put the illuminator probe under the patient's palm. His hand will appear red and the veins black.

• *What's the patient's condition?* Avoid veins in infected, injured, or irritated areas. The added stress of venipuncture may cause complications. Remember, if the patient's positioned on his side, choose a venipuncture site on the other side of his body.

• *How old is the patient?* You've probably decided that the best venipuncture site for Mr. Olson is on his hand or lower arm. But if your patient were an infant, your choice would be different, because protecting the needle from dislodgement is difficult. You'd probably choose a scalp vein since it's accessible and easy to protect. (Find out more about infant venipuncture on page 46.) However, within the first 24 to 72 hours after birth, the umbilical vein's an alternative site. (For more on umbilical catheters, see page 148.)

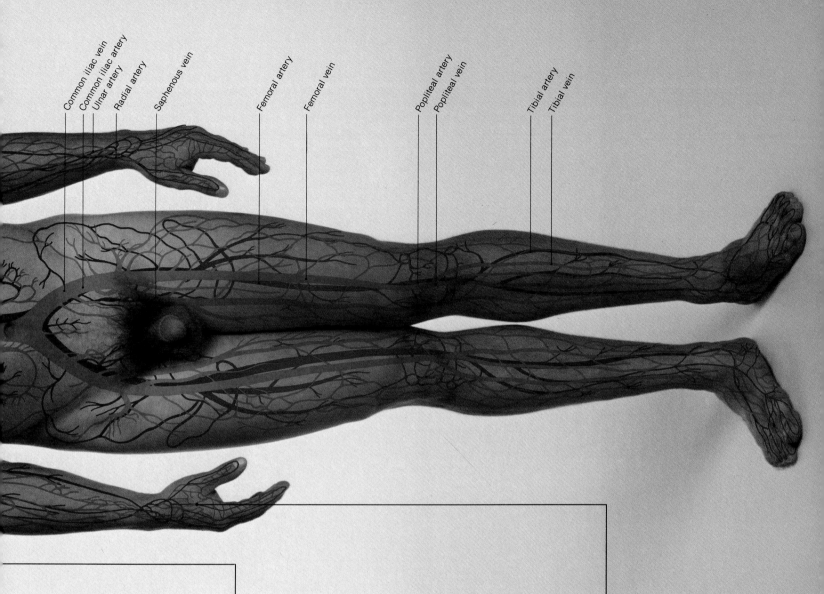

Common iliac vein
Common iliac artery
Ulnar artery
Radial artery
Saphenous vein
Femoral artery
Femoral vein
Popliteal artery
Popliteal vein
Tibial artery
Tibial vein

Antecubital fossa area

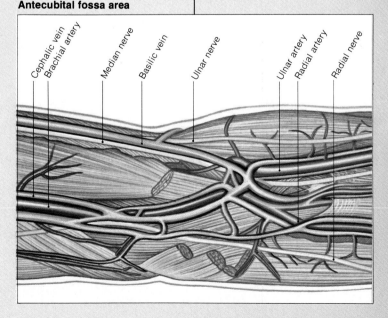

Cephalic vein
Brachial artery
Median nerve
Basilic vein
Ulnar nerve
Ulnar artery
Radial artery
Radial nerve

Dorsum of the hand

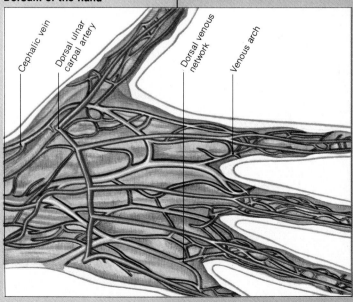

Cephalic vein
Dorsal ulnar carpal artery
Dorsal venous network
Venous arch

Venipuncture

Using the antecubital fossa for venipuncture

We've pictured a close-up view of the antecubital fossa on the preceding page. Because the veins in this area are visible and easily accessible, the antecubital fossa has proven ideal for short-term use, such as taking blood samples or administering unit-dose drugs. But try to avoid it (or any other area over a patient's joint) for long-term I.V. therapy. Unless the joint's immobilized, the tubing could kink or the cannula could pistol in and out of the vein, damaging it. Although splinting the joint may solve this problem, such a measure is both uncomfortable and inconvenient for the patient.

Study the illustration again. As you can see, the median nerve and the brachial artery lie near the veins at this point. Take special care to avoid them. If you accidentally hit the nerve, your patient will feel more pain than he would during a successful venipuncture. Withdraw the needle, and try again at another site. To minimize the risk of striking the artery, always feel for a pulse before performing venipuncture. If you should mistakenly enter the artery, you'll know at once because the blood flow will probably force the syringe plunger up the barrel. Withdraw the needle, and immediately apply manual pressure with a 2" x 2" sterile gauze pad for at least 7 minutes. Otherwise, the artery may bleed into the joint, causing serious complications. Then, apply a pressure bandage. Remember to check it periodically.

How veins and arteries differ

As you can see in these illustrations, certain differences exist in the internal structure of veins and arteries. And at least one of these differences can affect the ease with which you perform venipuncture. Consider the valves that appear at regular intervals throughout each vein, for example. If you hit a valve when you're inserting a catheter, you may have to withdraw the catheter and perform venipuncture in another vein. As an alternative, some hospitals will allow you to coil and tape down the part of the catheter which remains outside the skin. Know your hospital's policy before you perform venipuncture.

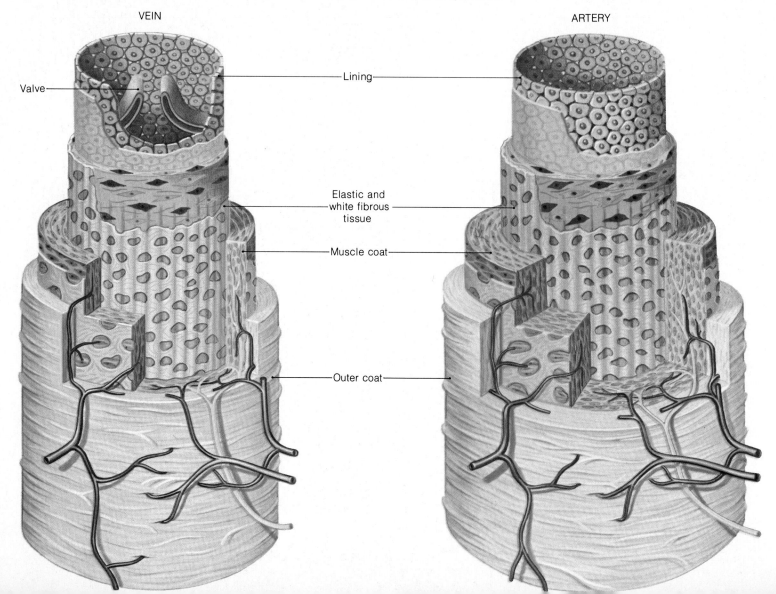

VEIN

ARTERY

Valve

Lining

Elastic and white fibrous tissue

Muscle coat

Outer coat

How to dilate a vein

1 *Planning venipuncture? As you know, you'll need to dilate the patient's vein before you can insert the needle or cannula.* To accomplish this, start by applying digital pressure just above the selected insertion site. If the patient's veins are large and prominent, this action will raise a vein quickly.

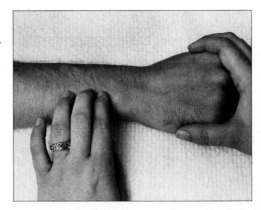

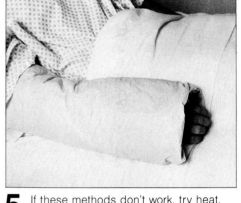

2 Now, apply a tourniquet made from a length of soft rubber tubing, or a wide strip of rubber tied in a slip knot, as shown in this photo. Or, if you prefer, use a blood pressure cuff. Place the tourniquet 2" to 6" above the site you've selected for venipuncture. Tuck part of the patient's gown sleeve under the tourniquet so his skin isn't pinched. Apply enough pressure to impede venous flow without stopping arterial flow. If arterial perfusion's maintained, you'll be able to feel the radial pulse.
📧 *Nursing tip:* For an infant or a thin adult, use a wide rubber band as a tourniquet.

5 If these methods don't work, try heat. Wrap the entire limb in warm wet towels for 10 to 20 minutes before you attempt venipuncture. Sustain the heat by wrapping the toweling in a bedsaver or a plastic bag. Then, when the veins are engorged, apply a tourniquet.

Remember, you can substitute a heating pad for wet toweling, if you wish. Or use an electric hair dryer to heat a site where a tourniquet can't be applied. But take care not to burn the skin, especially if the patient's unconscious. Put your own hand next to the selected site as you apply heat on it so you can tell immediately if it's getting too hot. Remember, don't use a hair dryer where the potential for fire or explosion exists; for example, near an oxygen tent.

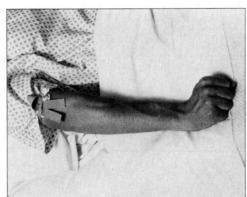

3 If applying a tourniquet doesn't do the trick, have the patient open and close his fist repeatedly, as this photo shows. Then, ask him to close his fist as you insert the needle and to open it again when the needle's in place. Remove the tourniquet.
📧 *Nursing tip:* If the selected vein's in one of the patient's extremities, it may help to place the limb below heart level for several minutes.

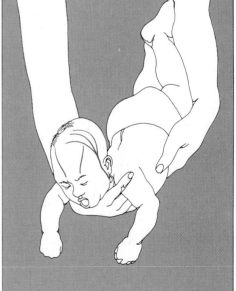

4 Suppose your patient's too feeble to clench and unclench his fist energetically. Apply a second tourniquet over his wrist, as we show here. Or, try applying the second tourniquet over his hand instead.

Here are two other ways to help raise a vein: With your fingers, tap or slap it lightly. Or place your fingers over the vein between the tourniquet and the venipuncture site, and use short, stroking motions to milk it down against the blood flow.

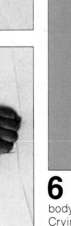

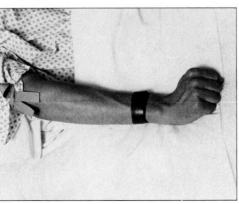

6 To dilate an infant's scalp veins, place his head lower than the rest of his body, which usually will make him cry. Crying, along with the lowered head position, will help raise his scalp veins.

Venipuncture

How to prep the skin

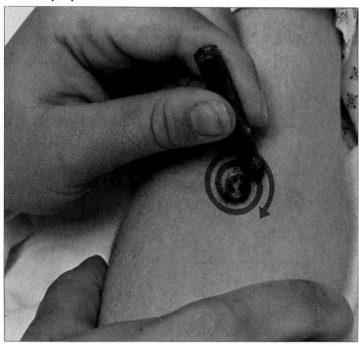

Venipuncture always poses an infection risk to the patient. To prevent or reduce this possibility, your first step must be to decrease skin bacteria with a thorough skin prep.

To save time, apply the tourniquet first, so the vein dilates while you do the prep. Unless the needle's larger than 18G, don't use a local anesthetic—it may trigger vein constriction and tissue swelling, making venipuncture harder. And don't shave the skin. Shaving may cause microabrasions, exposing skin tissue to bacteria. The antiseptic will clean the hair as well as the skin.

Here's how to clean the skin effectively:
• Select one of the skin preps described in the chart below. Most preps come prepackaged, complete with disposable applicators. (*Note:* Make sure the prep's room temperature before you begin. Cold antiseptic will cause the vein to constrict.)
• Apply the antiseptic to the skin with a circular motion, beginning at the intended venipuncture site and working outward. Cover an area about 2" in diameter. Then, return to the center and repeat the process. Continue the action for about 1 minute. (*Note:* Don't wave your hands above the skin to dry it—you'll increase the chance of contamination.)

Important: Read the following chart carefully for specific details on several common preps.

Nurses' guide to common skin preps

Antiseptic	Advantages	Disadvantages	Special considerations
iodine solution 2%, tincture 2%	• Kills bacteria, fungi, viruses, protozoa, and yeasts • Inexpensive and reliable	• May burn or chap skin • May cause an allergic reaction • Discolors skin	• Always ask the patient if he has any allergies before applying. • Wash off the iodine with 70% alcohol after 30 seconds. • Don't cover the skin before the iodine is washed off. • Don't mix iodine with hydrogen peroxide. • Sodium thiosulfate is the antidote of choice for accidental ingestion.
povidone-iodine (water-soluble complexes of iodine and organic compounds; also called iodophors) Betadine*, Proviodine**, Sepp	• Less irritating than iodine tinctures or solutions • Doesn't stain skin as much as iodine	• Less effective than regular iodine solutions • May be absorbed through the skin during prolonged use • May cause an allergic reaction	• Always ask the patient if he has any allergies before applying. • Do *not* wash it off—use full strength.
ethyl alcohol alcohol 70%, ethanol	• Effective as a fat solvent and germicidal when used in concentrations of 70% to 80% • May be used as a substitute prep when the patient's allergic to iodine	• Not effective against spore-forming organisms, viruses, or tubercle bacilli • Evaporates quickly • Flammable and explosive • Dries skin excessively	• If ethyl alcohol's unavailable, for whatever reason, don't use isopropyl alcohol as a substitute. It causes vasodilation, making bleeding more likely.

*Available in the United States and in Canada.
**Available only in Canada.

How to insert a winged-tip needle

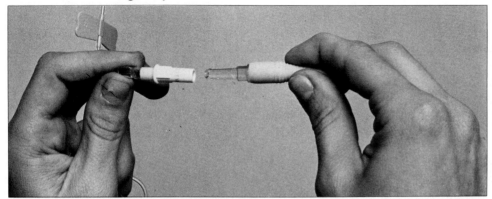

1 *Suppose you've already washed your hands, gathered the necessary equipment, and explained venipuncture to the patient. Now you're ready to insert the needle into his vein. Because you'll probably be using a winged-tip needle, we've chosen to feature it in this photostory. To find out how to insert it properly—using the easy, indirect method—study the following photos:*

First, spike the container as we explained on page 16. Then, attach the tubing adapter to the needle connector, as we show in this photo.

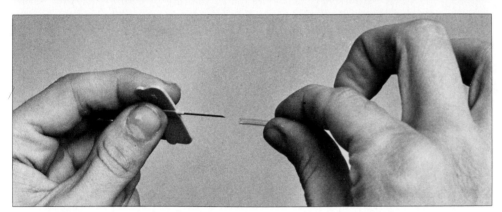

2 Flush both the tubing and the needle with fluid to remove air. Clamp the tube to stop fluid flow, and recap the needle, as shown, to maintain sterility.

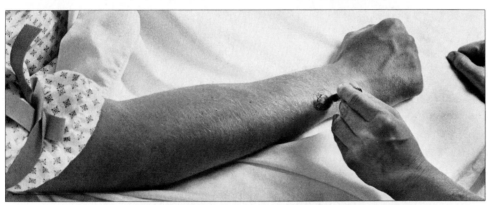

3 Select a vein, and apply a tourniquet, using the technique described earlier in this section. Prep the skin around the insertion site, as the nurse is doing in this photo.

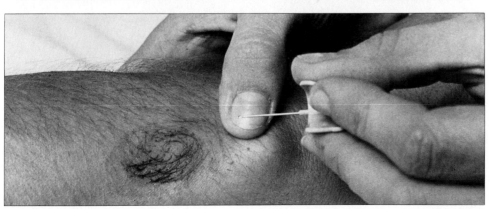

4 After the vein's dilated, stabilize it by anchoring it with your thumb and stretching the skin downward, as shown here. If the vein's in the patient's hand, you may find it helps to flex his wrist. Or ask the patient to help stabilize his vein by first making a fist with his free hand, then clasping it with the hand you're about to puncture.

Venipuncture

How to insert a winged-tip needle continued

5 When you've completed these steps, remove the needle cap. Point the needle in the direction of the blood flow and hold it at a 45° angle above the skin, with the bevel facing up. Now, you're ready to insert the needle into the vein, using what's commonly called the indirect method of venipuncture.

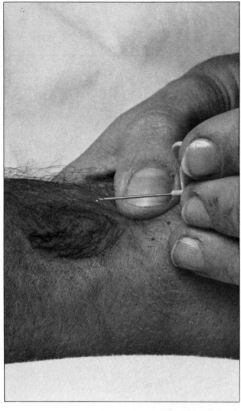

7 Now, decrease the needle angle until the needle's almost level with the skin surface, and direct it toward the vein you've selected. You'll feel very little resistance as the needle goes through subcutaneous tissue; you'll feel considerably more resistance when you reach the vein.

Proceeding carefully, attempt to puncture the vein with the needle. To confirm that you've punctured the vein, watch for blood backflow in the tubing. For more details on blood backflow, see page 34.

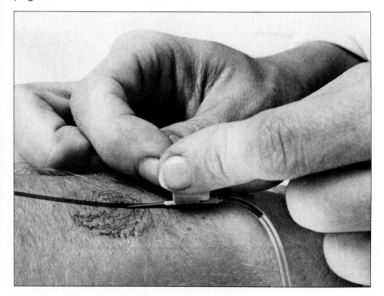

8 Continue to advance the needle until it's well within the vein. By exerting a gentle, lifting pressure during this step, you can keep the needle from piercing the opposite wall of the vein.

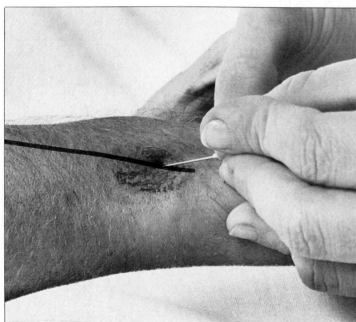

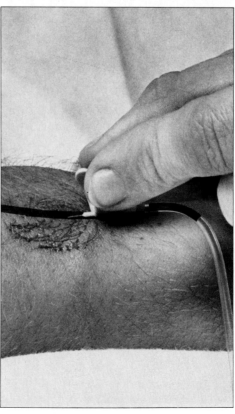

6 Here's how to do it: Pinch the wings together tightly, as the nurse is doing in this photo. Keeping your hand steady, pierce the patient's skin at a point slightly to one side of the vein, about ½" below the spot where you plan to puncture the vein wall.
🕮 *Nursing tip:* To reduce the patient's discomfort during this step, ask him to inhale at the exact moment the needle enters his skin.

9 Now, you're ready to begin the infusion. Remove the tourniquet from the patient's arm, open the flow clamp in the tubing, and check for free flow. Then, partially close the clamp until you've securely taped the needle and tubing.

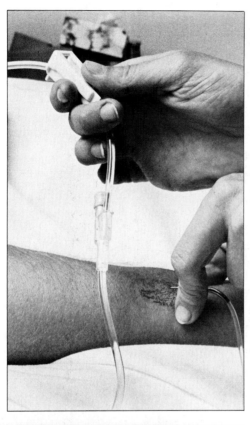

11 Now, place another strip of tape perpendicular to the first two. Either put it directly on top of the wings, or put it just below the wings, directly on top of the tubing. Depending on the site's location, use whichever way lends more stability.

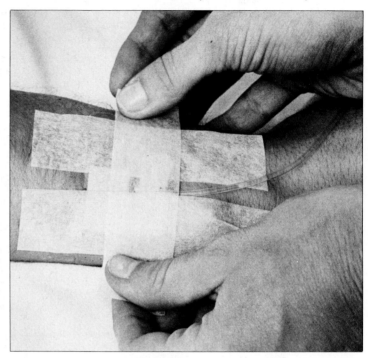

12 If you prefer, do as the nurse is doing here. Use the H method of taping to stabilize the needle *before* you apply the antimicrobial ointment and the 2" x 2" sterile gauze pad. This way, you can examine the site just by removing the bandage.

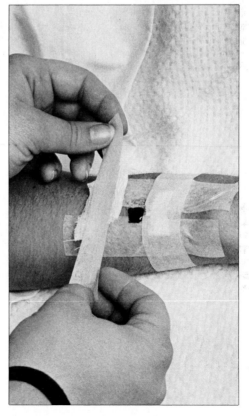

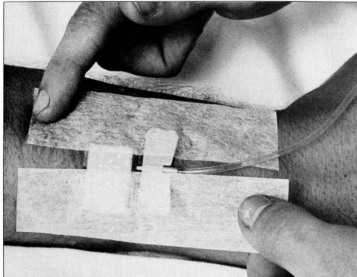

10 Apply antimicrobial ointment at the venipuncture site, and cover it with an adhesive bandage. Is your patient allergic to adhesive? Use a 2" x 2" sterile gauze pad instead. Remember, if you prefer, you can apply the ointment to the dressing rather than to the patient's skin.

Whatever type dressing you use, be sure to securely tape it in place. To tape using the H method, place one strip of tape over each wing, keeping the tape parallel to the needle. But remember, the tape's not sterile. Don't let it contaminate the site.

Venipuncture

How to insert a winged-tip needle continued

13 Next, loop the tubing, and secure it with more tape, as shown here. Because a loop gives the tubing more play, the needle's less likely to become dislodged if the tubing is accidentally pulled. However, don't make the loop so small that you kink it and restrict the fluid flow.

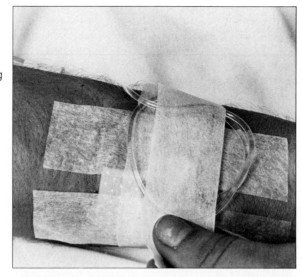

14 When you've completed this, use a watch to set the flow rate. Remember, to flow at the proper rate, an I.V. container must hang 30" to 36" (1 m) above the insertion site.

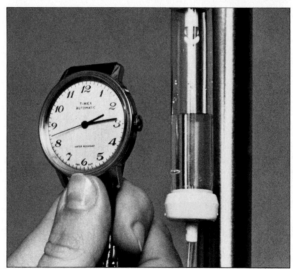

15 Finally, label the site with the necessary information. To do this properly, cut a strip of tape and place it on a flat surface. On it, write the following data: date and time of insertion, type and gauge of needle, and your initials. Place it over the dressing. *Important:* Never label the tape *after* you've placed it on the dressing; doing so will irritate the venipuncture site.

When you've completed the dressing label, make sure the container and tubing are labeled properly. Document the entire procedure in your notes. To find out how to do this correctly, see page 43.

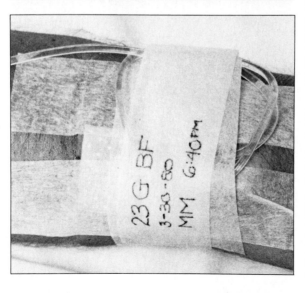

How to check needle placement

The best way to tell whether or not you've correctly entered the vein is by checking for a blood backflow. The procedure's simple. Lower the I.V. container below the venipuncture site. Bend the tubing at a point several inches away from the needle or cannula and then release it. If the needle's properly placed in the vein, gravity will usually pull blood into the tubing.

But backflow's not a foolproof indication of correct placement. You might get a backflow when the needle or cannula's only partly in the vein. In this case, the flow rate will be sluggish when you begin the infusion. If this happens, slightly advance the needle or cannula, and check the flow rate again. You may also get a backflow when the needle or cannula's passed through the vein and out the opposite wall. But then, the backflow will be minimal. If you try for backflow after a moment, you won't get any.

On the other hand, the absence of backflow doesn't always mean the needle or cannula's outside the vein. A tourniquet that's too tight may be causing the problem. Loosen it and see what happens. You may also not get a backflow when you're using a small vein, or when your patient's elderly or has low blood pressure. In such cases, try drawing blood with a needle and syringe in the tubing port. Pinch off the tubing above the port, insert the needle, and draw back on the plunger. *Remember:* Pinch off the tubing first, so you don't aspirate I.V. fluid instead of blood.

Maybe you're not getting a backflow because the needle or cannula's pressed against the opposite wall of the vein and is blocked. If you suspect that's happened—and you're using a winged-tip needle—pull the needle back slightly. If you're using an INC or an ONC, withdraw the needle first. Then, pull the catheter back slightly. Both procedures should unblock the needle or cannula tip and permit backflow.

After the infusion's begun, you can make sure the needle or catheter's in the vein by applying a tourniquet just above the entry site. This'll occlude the vein and stop the infusion flow. If the flow continues, the needle or catheter's not properly placed. Stop the infusion immediately, and withdraw the needle or catheter. In this case, fluid may be infiltrating surrounding tissue. The surest sign of infiltration is swelling and coolness at the entry site. Check the site frequently. At the first sign of infiltration, stop the infusion and remove the needle or catheter.

Document what you've done.

Inserting a needle: The direct method

1 On page 32, we showed you how to do venipuncture by approaching the vein indirectly, about ½" below the point where you plan to penetrate the vein wall. But now, we'll show you a more direct approach. It requires considerably more skill than the indirect method, but it's worth learning because it's less painful for the patient when done correctly.

Note: Always use this method when doing venipuncture on an infant. You'll find that it makes it easier to insert a short needle into a tiny vein.

Start by dilating the vein and prepping the skin, as described before. Hold the needle at a 30° angle over the vein, and point it in the direction of the blood flow.

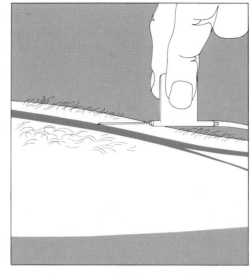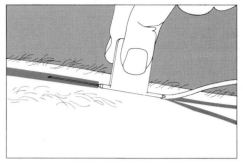

2 Now, with one quick motion, pierce the skin with the needle and advance it into the vein. To confirm a successful vein puncture, check for blood backflow. Then, remove the tourniquet, and secure the needle and tubing with either the H method, explained earlier, or the other methods which follow.

How to position the bevel

1 *On page 32, we explained how to insert a winged-tip needle with the bevel facing up. As you know, this position usually causes less trauma to the vein and is less painful for the patient. But sometimes the bevel-down position's better. Here's why:* The illustration to the right shows what a needle in the *bevel-up* position looks like when it enters a vein. If the needle and the vein have approximately the same diameter, this position's likely to perforate the vein's opposite wall on insertion and cause a hematoma. As you can see in the illustration below, the bevel-down position is less likely to cause this problem.

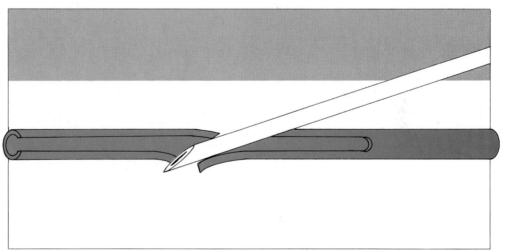

2 In this illustration, you'll see still another reason why the bevel-down position sometimes is better. As you know, entering a vein successfully doesn't guarantee that the vein won't collapse and block the bevel when you remove the tourniquet. In that case, manipulating the needle slightly within the vein may relieve the blockage. But if you try this with a needle in the bevel-up position, you run a greater risk of perforating the vein's opposite wall. So when you enter a relatively small vein with a large-bore (20G or larger) needle, use the bevel-down position.

Remember, a needle that's properly placed in a superficial vein is usually palpable. If you can't feel the needle tip easily, you've probably gone through the vein. Remove the needle immediately.

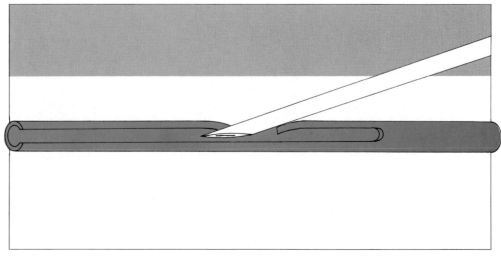

Venipuncture

Taping a winged-tip needle: The U method

1 *The photos on page 33 show you how to tape the winged-tip needle using the H method. Now, we'll illustrate two alternate ways: the U method and the chevron method. All three methods are effective. However, you'll probably find that one's more stable than the others, depending on where the venipuncture site's located.*

Here's how to do the U taping method. As soon as you've completed venipuncture, apply antimicrobial ointment to the site, as the nurse has done here.

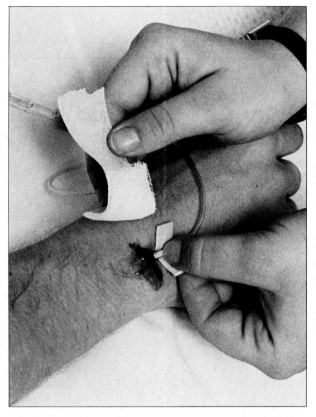

2 Then, tape a 2" x 2" sterile gauze pad over the site. (If you prefer, use an adhesive bandage strip instead, but make sure your patient isn't allergic to the tape on the strip.)

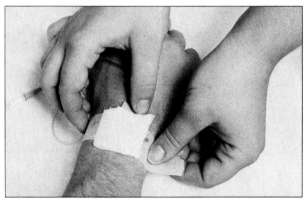

3 Now, cut three strips of ¼" tape. Keeping the sticky side up, place one strip under the tubing, parallel to the wings. *Remember:* The tape's not sterile. Don't let it contaminate the site.

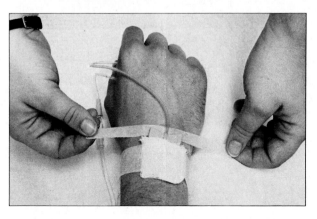

4 Bring each side of the tape up over the wing, folding it over on itself, as shown here. Press it down over each wing at a 90° angle.

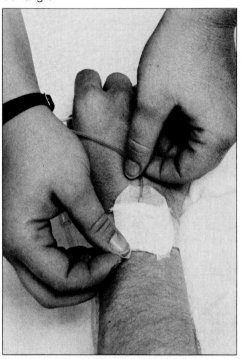

5 Finally, loop the tubing, and secure it with the second piece of tape. Mark your last piece of tape with the date and time of insertion, type and gauge of needle, and your initials. Then, apply it to the dressing. Document exactly what you've done.

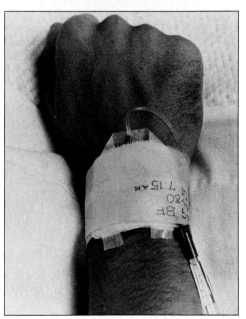

Taping a winged-tip needle: The chevron method

1 *Now, we'll show how to do the chevron, or criss-cross, method of taping. Study these photos closely. You can use this method to secure both over-the-needle (ONC) catheters and inside-the-needle (INC) catheters.*

Begin by applying antimicrobial ointment to the site as soon as you've completed venipuncture. Then, cover the site with an adhesive bandage strip or a 2" x 2" sterile gauze pad. Apply a short strip of ¼" tape across both wings.

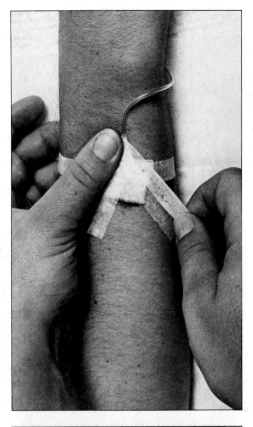

3 Cross each end of the tape over the opposite wing, so the tape sticks to both wings and the patient's skin. Then, for added security, apply the second strip of tape the same way. Make sure it overlaps the first, as shown here.

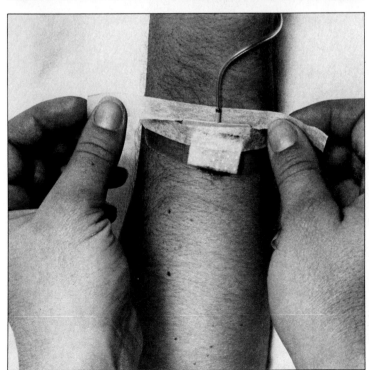

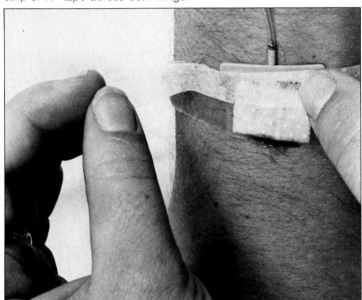

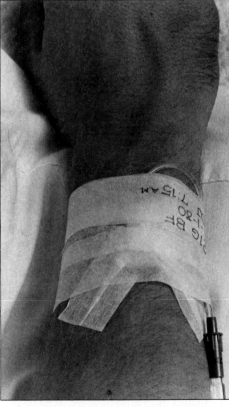

4 Finally, loop and secure the tubing to the dressing with tape. Mark your last piece of tape with the following information: date and time of insertion, type and gauge of needle, and your initials. Document what you've done.

2 Next, cut two long strips of ¼" tape. Place one of them sticky-side up under the tubing, parallel to the wings. ☎ *Nursing tip:* For convenience, cut all the tape you need before beginning.

Venipuncture

TROUBLESHOOTING

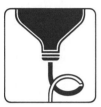

How to solve taping problems

What if you're securing a winged-tip needle and the adhesive tape won't stick to the patient's skin? Then try these tips:
• Shave or clip excess hair around the insertion site. The tape will adhere better to the skin, and removing it won't hurt as much. However, don't let the clippings contaminate the venipuncture site.
• Use paper tape, remembering to thoroughly dry damp or clammy skin first.
• Apply tincture of benzoin, again remembering to dry the skin first. Wait for the benzoin to dry long enough to become sticky. Then tape.

Inserting an over-the-needle catheter

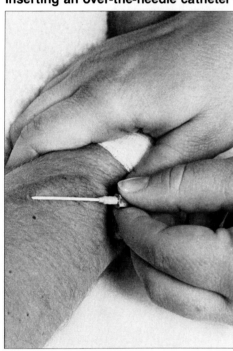

1 *The initial steps for inserting an over-the-needle catheter (ONC) are the same as for inserting a winged-tip needle. Turn back to pages 31 and 32, and review steps 1 through 8 for winged-tip insertion. Then, follow the same procedure to place the ONC securely in the vein. After you've checked for blood backflow, follow these steps to complete the procedure.*

As the above photo shows, have a 4" x 4" sterile gauze pad ready to slip under the hub as soon as the cannula's in place. (If you prefer, use a skin prep swab instead.) This provides a firm, sterile field for the connection point, and protects the hub and adapter from touch contamination. It'll also catch any blood that spills when you withdraw the needle. Of course, if it becomes soiled, remove it after you connect the hub and adapter.

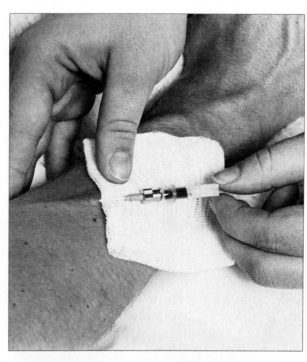

2 Next, hold the needle hub firmly in place with your thumb and forefinger. Now, advance the cannula another ¼", to make sure it's in the vein properly. Why? Because the catheter's slightly shorter than the needle. As a result, blood backflow sometimes occurs when the needle alone is in the vein. The extra ¼" advancement provides added assurance that the cannula's correctly placed. *Important:* If you feel any resistance, don't force the catheter. Instead, withdraw the needle and catheter *together.* If you try to withdraw the catheter first, you may cut it on the needle's sharp bevel, causing a catheter embolism. Then, attempt venipuncture again at another site.

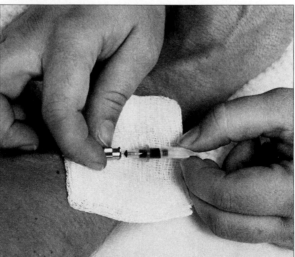

3 When you're sure the cannula's placed correctly, release the tourniquet. Now you're ready to withdraw the needle. If the needle sticks inside the catheter, grasp the catheter hub firmly, and rotate the needle to loosen it.

4 As you remove the needle, press lightly on the skin over the catheter tip to prevent bleeding, as shown here.

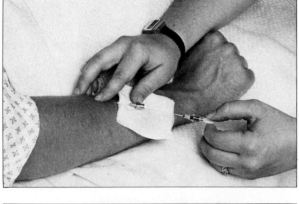

5 Now, connect the adapter of the administration set to the catheter hub. As you do, keep your finger pressed against the catheter tip.

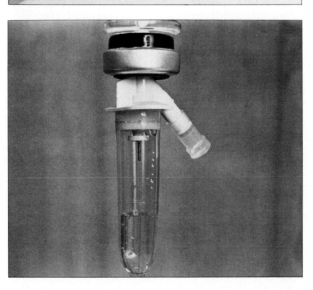

6 When you've completed the connection, let the I.V. fluid flow freely for a few seconds to assure proper placement of the catheter. Then, set a slow flow rate until you finish dressing and taping the site.

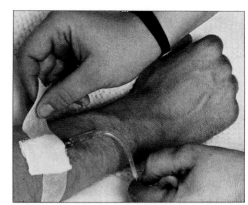

7 Apply antimicrobial ointment and a fresh 2" x 2" sterile gauze pad or adhesive bandage over the venipuncture site.

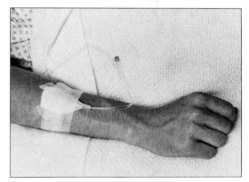

8 Secure the catheter with the chevron taping method, explained on page 37. Make sure the tape covers both the hub and the adapter. Then, use a second piece of tape to anchor the 2" x 2" sterile gauze pad over the insertion site. *Important:* Don't wrap the tape completely around the patient's arm. Doing so could restrict blood flow and produce edema.

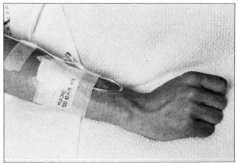

9 When you've accomplished these steps, loop the tubing loosely enough to avoid kinking, and tape it securely. Remember to mark the tape clearly with the date and time of insertion, type and gauge of ONC, and your initials. Then, adjust the flow rate, and document the procedure.

Venipuncture

Inserting an inside-the-needle catheter

1 *Inserting an inside-the-needle catheter (INC) is a little different from inserting an ONC. The following photos will show you how it's done.*

Examine the INC in this photo. As you can see, we've separated the parts so you can distinguish them easily. Of course, before you begin venipuncture, you'd only loosen them.

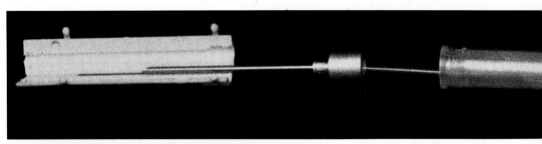

2 Next, apply a tourniquet to the patient's arm. Since the catheter's fairly long (usually 8"), make sure the tourniquet's well above the venipuncture site. Otherwise, it'll block your efforts to advance the catheter.

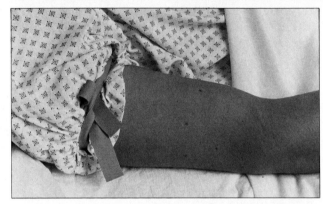

3 Now, you're ready to insert the INC into the patient's vein. The procedure is the same as for inserting a winged-tip needle. Review steps 1 through 8 on pages 31 and 32.

As soon as the cannula's in the vein, watch for blood backflow into the collar, as shown here. When you're sure the needle's properly placed, push the flow control plug into the female adapter, to prevent the blood from spilling out of the catheter. As you can see, we've already completed this step in the photo.

4 Now, you're ready to advance the catheter into the vein. Here's how: First, grasp the hub with one hand to stabilize the needle. With your other hand, grasp the catheter through the protective plastic sleeve. (Holding the catheter through the sleeve prevents contamination.) Gently push the catheter part of the way into the vein.

Then, hold the catheter between your finger and thumb to keep it in place. Move your other hand back to its original position, and slide the catheter forward again. Repeat the process until the entire catheter's inserted. *Note:* If you encounter resistance while advancing the catheter, try removing the tourniquet. But if the catheter *still* won't move easily, don't force it. Instead, withdraw the needle and catheter together, as we describe on page 42, and make a second attempt at another site.

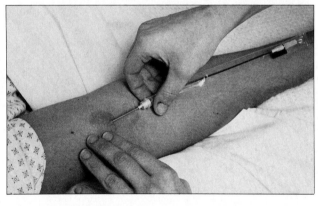

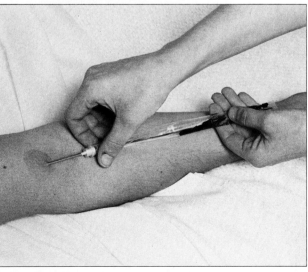

5 If you haven't already done so, remove the tourniquet as soon as the catheter's fully advanced. Gently press a 2" x 2" sterile gauze pad on the vein (to hold the catheter in place), and withdraw the needle. Maintain pressure over the site for 1 minute after withdrawing the needle, to prevent a hematoma.

6 This photo shows a bevel cover, sometimes called a needle protector. It prevents the needle bevel from cutting the patient or the catheter. Place the needle midway in the channel of the bevel cover, making sure that the catheter also lies in the channel. Then, snap the bevel cover shut.

7 Grasp the bevel cover near the hub. With your other hand, remove the collar.

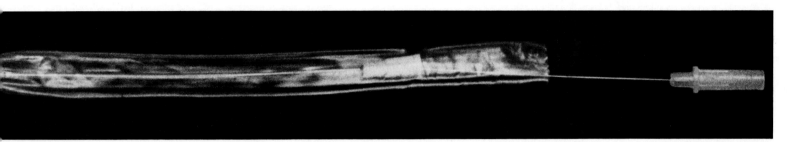

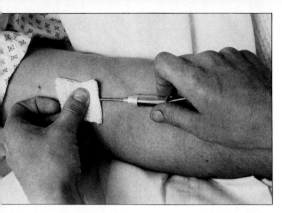

8 Next, grasp the hub firmly with one hand. With the other hand, slide the bevel cover back along the catheter until it clicks firmly into the hub. *Nursing tip:* If the catheter's not yet fully advanced, you may prefer to continue advancing the catheter until the hub meets the bevel cover and clicks in place.

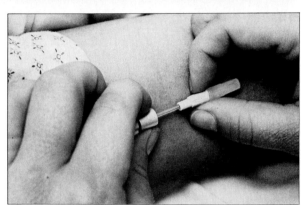

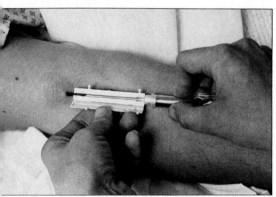

9 Put a 2" x 2" sterile gauze pad beneath the hub to catch any spilled blood. Hold the I.V. tubing between your fingers so you can connect it quickly. Then, remove the flow control adapter and obturator, as shown here.

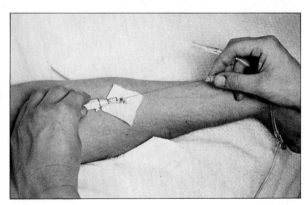

10 Now, attach the catheter hub to the infusion adapter. Open the infusion flow control, check for free flow, and reduce the flow rate while you secure the catheter.

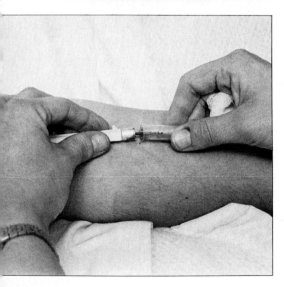

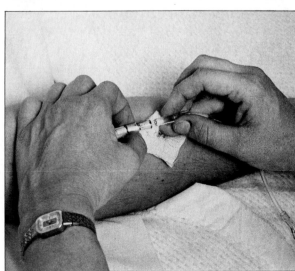

Venipuncture

Inserting an inside-the-needle catheter continued

11 Apply antimicrobial ointment to the venipuncture site. Then, cover it with an adhesive bandage or a 2" x 2" sterile gauze pad, and secure with tape. *Remember:* The tape's not sterile. Don't let it contaminate the site.

Secure the catheter near the injection site with the chevron method of taping, explained on page 37. Then, tape the bevel cover, needle/hub connection, and tubing to the skin. Mark the tape clearly with the date and time of insertion, the gauge of the catheter, and your initials. Finally, adjust the flow rate, and document the procedure.

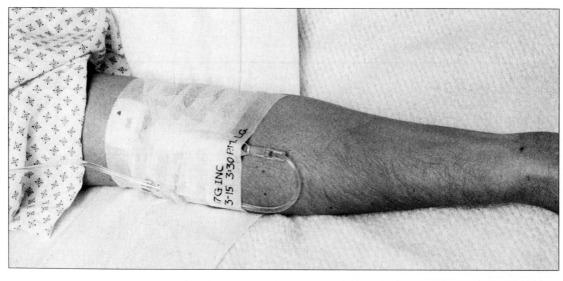

12 Sometimes special problems occur; for example, the bevel cover may be misplaced or contaminated. If that happens, tape a sterile tongue blade under the needle to stabilize it.

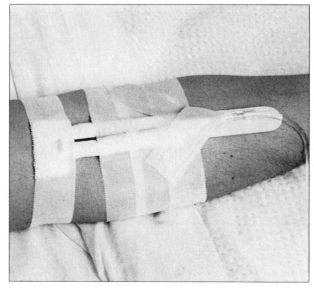

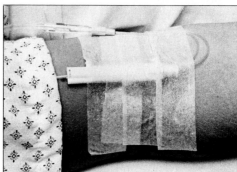

13 Or, suppose you encounter resistance while advancing a catheter in an emergency. You may not have time to withdraw the INC and start over. In this situation, withdraw and secure the needle as you would if the catheter were fully advanced. Then, loop and tape the excess catheter and tubing, as shown in this photo.

TROUBLESHOOTING

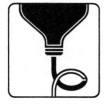

Coping with I.V. catheter insertion problems

How should a catheter enter the vein? In a word, smoothly. If you feel resistance and you're using a relatively long catheter, try removing the tourniquet. Doing this will open the vein and restore blood flow. Now the catheter should move easily.

But if it still doesn't, don't force it. Instead, withdraw the needle and catheter *together*. Don't withdraw the catheter first, because you could cut it on the needle bevel and create a catheter embolus. Once you've withdrawn the needle and catheter, apply gentle pressure to the site. Then, tape a 2" x 2" sterile gauze pad over it to prevent hematoma.

If possible, use the patient's other arm for the next attempt. Why? Because placing a tourniquet above the first site increases the risk of hematoma. However, if you must use the same arm again, avoid selecting a vein flowing into the vein you first chose. When the tourniquet's reapplied, it may cause some blood to ooze from the old site. Be prepared for it by gently pressing a gauze pad over the site to minimize bleeding.

How to document I.V. therapy

Documenting I.V. therapy doesn't stop with labeling the dressing; you must label the container and tubing too. In addition, you must also chart all I.V. procedures as well as your own observations of the patient's condition.

How to label the container

The manufacturer's label identifies the solution in the container and its expiration date; always read it carefully. Now, write this information on a second label:
• Patient's name, I.D. number, and room number
• Dosage and absorption time
• Drip rate
• Date and time the container was hung
• Container number. The National Coordinating Committee of Large Volume Parenterals (NCCLVP) recommends that you number each container sequen-

tially, regardless of how many days I.V. therapy lasts. For example, if 3,000 ml of solution are ordered on May 10, 1980, this day's 1,000 ml bottles are numbered 1, 2, 3. If 3,000 ml more are ordered on May 11, these bottles are numbered 4, 5, 6. This system minimizes administration errors.
• Your name.

Now, as shown below, apply the label upside down so you can read it when the container's hanging on the pole. Make sure it doesn't cover the name of the solution printed at the top of the manufacturer's bottle. Finally, apply a timing label, which we'll explain how to prepare on the next page.

If you administer an admixture, apply a label identifying the additive. Follow the same format as above. If the additive has a short life (stability), include its expiration time.

How to label the tubing

Always label I.V. tubing to make sure it's changed every 48 hours. Use a different colored tape for each day of the week as a handy reference. Or, simply wrap a strip of tape around the tubing, leaving a tab. Mark the date and time the tubing was last changed on the tab. If you're using more than one tubing (when you're adding another container, for example), label each separately.

How to chart I.V. procedures

Document each venipuncture completely. Your nurses' notes should include:
• Date and time of venipuncture
• Amount and type of solution, including additives
• Dosage and absorption time
• Drip rate
• Container number
• Type and gauge of needle or

cannula set
• Insertion site
• Patient's condition
• Your name.

Suppose an infusion's running when you start your shift. Check things out, and chart your observations of the patient's condition and the venipuncture site. Describe any complications and the actions you took to remedy them. If you notice swelling, for example, measure the area it covers, and describe the skin color so the nurse on the next shift can compare findings.

If you add medication to an infusion, chart that too. Each entry should include the information listed above, except for date and time of venipuncture and the type and gauge of the cannula, which you needn't repeat.

Remember: Don't rely on your observations alone. Ask the patient how he feels.

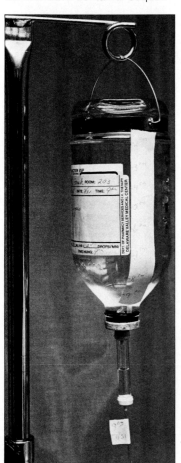

				NAME *Jones, Thomas*
				AGE *52*

Patient Progress Notes

DATE	TIME	NO.	PROBLEM	
12/31/79	3 P.M.	3	Hypokalemia	S: Patient complains of muscle weakness, nausea, and vomiting.
				O: Pulse 52 and regular, respirations 20. Vomited x 1-250ml of bile-colored liquid. Skin warm and dry.
				A: Need for hydration and potassium replacement.
				P: Monitor I & O carefully. Check I.V. insertion site for signs of infiltration. Redress site 1/1/80. See Care Plan.
				I: 20g. Jelco with in-line filter inserted in the Ⓛ antecubital space at 10:30 A.M. #2 bottle of 1000ml. of D₅W with 40meq of KCl added, hung and running at 21gtts/min. Intake 350ml. Output: 500ml. straw-colored urine and 250ml of bile-colored vomitus.
				Jean Francis, RN

Venipuncture

How to make a timing label

1 *Preparing a timing label should be an important part of your labeling routine. Why? Because a properly prepared timing label lets you see at a glance whether or not the solution's running at the prescribed rate.* Although these labels are available commercially, you can easily make one by placing a strip of adhesive tape vertically on the container, as shown here. On the tape, write the approximate time the solution level should reach each volume mark on the container. At the bottom of the label, write the time the container should be empty. If the solution's running too quickly or too slowly, adjust the flow rate. Don't forget to document the procedure.

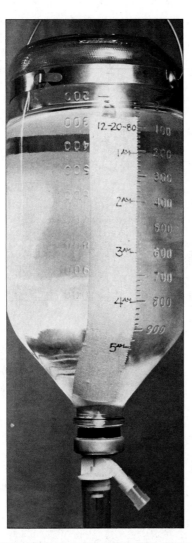

Hourly flow rate

10	5	8	6	12

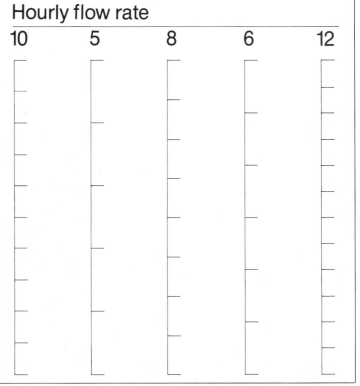

2 The handy chart shown above will help you make timing labels quickly and accurately. On a piece of cardboard, mark off five columns showing flow rates for 1,000 ml delivered over 5 hours, 6 hours, 8 hours, 10 hours, and 12 hours (or whatever time periods are commonly ordered at your hospital). Cover the cardboard with transparent plastic or an overexposed X-ray, and tape it to your medicine cart or an accessible spot in the nurses' station. Then, whenever you need to make a timing label, you have a convenient and handy guide.

Applying splints and restraints

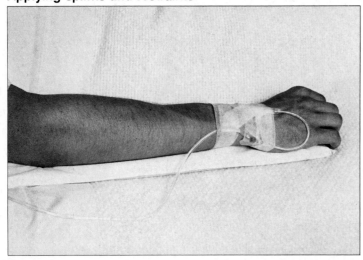

1 *When the venipuncture site's at a joint or if your patient's restless, consider applying a splint to stabilize the needle or catheter. Of course, if the patient's confused or combative, he may need the added protection of restraints. (However, don't apply restraints without a doctor's order.) The following photos will show you how to apply splints and restraints effectively.*
　Suppose you've decided to apply a splint. Which is better—a long or a short one? This depends on the location of the venipuncture site. You may find a short splint adequate when the site's on the hand or lower arm. But you'll need a long one to protect a site in the antecubital fossa. For the patient's comfort, pad the splint first. Then, position his arm with palm down to keep the body properly aligned and to prevent injury to the upper arm's nerves and muscles. Make sure the hand's supported by the end of the splint, as you see in this photo.
　📨 *Nursing tip:* In a pinch, you can fashion a splint from a rolled towel, a tissue box, or an I.V. tubing box. But since these improvisations won't hold up for an active patient, replace them with a splint as soon as possible.

Applying splints and restraints *continued*

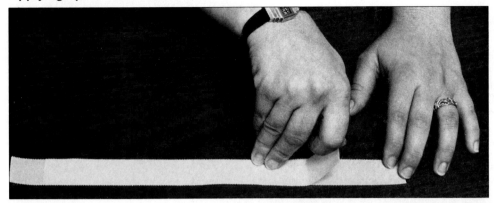

2 Now, you're ready to secure the splint. To insure free blood circulation and ease the eventual removal of the splint, you'll want to face, or backstrap, the adhesive securing the splint. To do this, first tear two strips of tape of equal width, one the diameter of the patient's arm and the other twice that length. Then, put the shorter piece in the center of the long one, with the sticky sides together. You should have about 5" of sticky tape left at each end. Prepare at least three of these faced tape strips if you're using a long splint, and two to secure a short one.

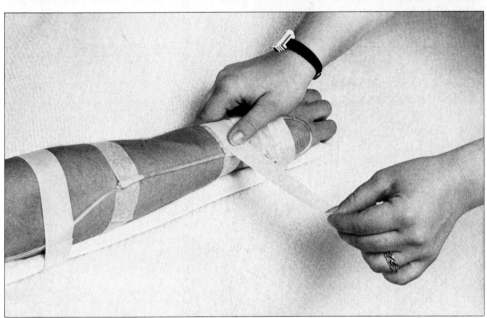

3 Now, wrap the tape around the arm and splint, keeping the faced part of the tape against the patient's arm and the sticky part against the splint. Take care not to impede circulation, but tape securely enough to immobilize the arm.
Nursing tip: As an alternative to taping the splint in the above manner, wrap gauze around both the splint and the arm, and tape over the gauze.

Don't tape over the venipuncture site. This way, you can easily remove the dressing to observe the site.

If the splint will be left in place for a long time, encourage the patient to exercise his hand periodically by squeezing a rubber ball or gauze roll.

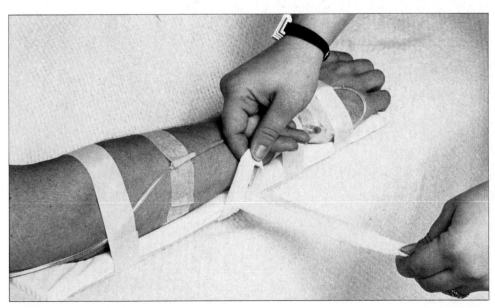

4 Suppose your patient's *very* restless, and the doctor's ordered restraints. Remember, the patient may be upset by the idea that he needs to be restrained, especially if he's become disoriented. Tactfully explain how restraints will help keep his I.V. line in place. Avoid using a judgmental tone; don't give the impression you're punishing him.

Although ready-made restraints are available, you can easily make one with a roll of gauze. Just slip the gauze under the patient's arm and around the splint, as shown here. *Important:* Don't tie the gauze to the patient's arm. It may act as a tourniquet, restricting circulation and clotting the catheter.

Venipuncture

Applying splints and restraints continued

5 Now, tie the other end of the restraint to the bed frame, toward the foot of the bed. *Note:* For safety's sake, don't tie the restraint to the bed's side rail. Make sure the knot's out of the patient's reach once the bed rail's raised. (For clarity, we've left the bed rail down in these photos.) Remember, a patient who needs restraints must never be left unattended with the bed rails down.

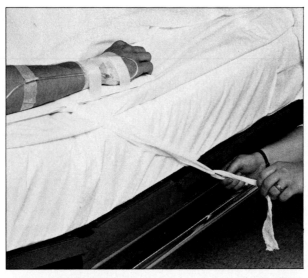

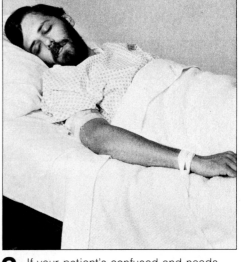

6 If both arms are restrained, keep the restraints short enough to keep the arms apart. But don't make them so short that the patient can't move at all. If the patient's turned on his side, adjust the restraints so his arms don't touch. Use a pillow to keep his arms apart, as shown here.

🕭 *Nursing tip:* For some patients you may need only a 2″ stockinette cover to protect the site. In such cases, cut a hole for the thumb, and bring the stockinette up over the I.V. site. Roll it back to inspect the site.

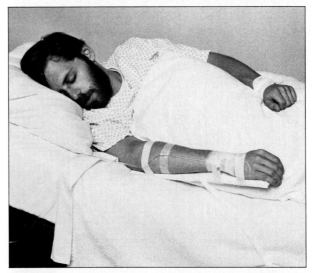

7 If the patient's a child or a confused adult, keep the flow clamp out of his reach. Running a strip of tape beneath the clamp will prevent him (or a meddlesome visitor) from pulling it down.

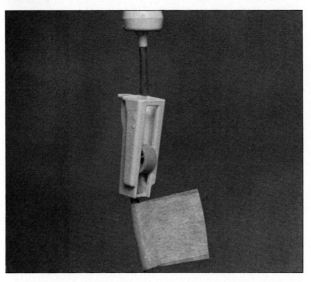

8 If your patient's confused and needs restraints, consider using the cephalic vein well above the antecubital fossa for a venipuncture site. Then the patient will have more freedom of movement, and the restraints won't interfere with the venipuncture site. To apply restraints, loop the gauze around his wrist, as shown in photo 4, and tie the other end to the bed frame.

Suppose the venipuncture site's on the hand or forearm. If you apply a restraint without splinting the arm, don't tie the gauze in such a way that the catheter presses down on the vein. This will irritate the vein and increase the risk of phlebitis.

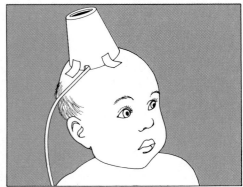

9 To protect a venipuncture site on an infant's scalp, put a stockinette on his head. Or, try this ingenious suggestion: Cut off the bottom of a small paper cup. Then, cut a small slot through the rim to accommodate the tubing. Place the cup over the needle so the tubing extends through the slot. Secure the cup with strips of tape, as shown here. The opening at the top of the cup lets you observe the site without disturbing it.

Replacing I.V. equipment

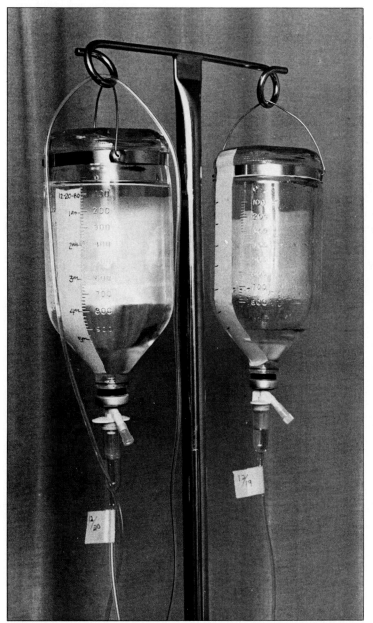

1 *How often should you change I.V. equipment? The Center for Disease Control, in Atlanta, recommends that you change needles, catheters, and tubing every 48 hours; and change bags, bottles, and dressings every 24 hours. Whenever possible, change the tubing and the container together. Remember, the more you handle the equipment, the greater the chance of contamination.*

Occasionally, you'll have to be flexible. For example, if your patient has few available veins left, you may have to leave a catheter in place longer than 48 hours. If so, be especially alert for signs of infection and infiltration.

On the following pages, you'll learn how to change the tubing and container together. As always, begin with a thorough hand washing.

Next, assemble a complete set of equipment, including tubing, container, dressings, and tape. Spike the container, prime the tubing, close the flow clamp, and cap the line as shown on page 16.

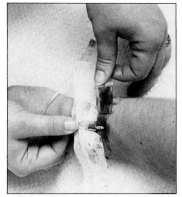

2 Now, you're ready to untape the old dressing. To avoid dislodging the needle or catheter as you work, hold the needle hub with one hand while you untape the dressing with the other hand. Then, ask the patient not to move unnecessarily until everything's retaped.

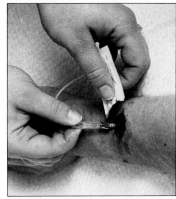

3 As soon as the dressing's removed, clean the skin around the venipuncture site with an iodine solution or an alcohol prep. Then, apply antimicrobial ointment, as shown here. To stabilize the catheter, put a fresh adhesive bandage or a 2" x 2" sterile gauze pad over the site.

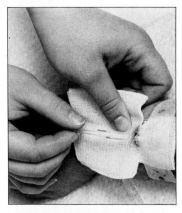

4 Close the flow clamp on the old tubing, and place a 4" x 4" sterile gauze pad under the hub to create a sterile field.

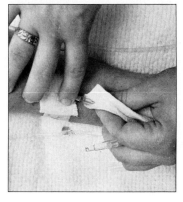

5 Now, press one of your fingers over the catheter to prevent bleeding, as the nurse is doing here. Grasp the hub with the sterile gauze pad to prevent touch contamination, and carefully disconnect the old adapter. If you hold the end of the new tubing between your fingers, as you see here, you can insert it quickly.

Venipuncture

Replacing I.V. equipment continued

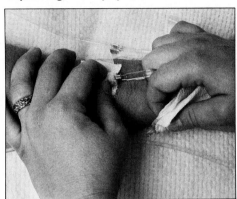

6 Remove the protective cap from the new tubing adapter. Working quickly, connect the adapter to the needle hub, as we show here.

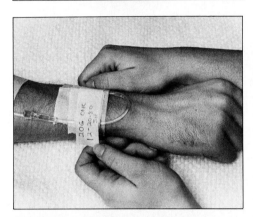

7 Secure the catheter, using the chevron method of taping described on page 37. Label the dressing, and readjust the flow rate. *Remember:* Don't write the label after it's on the patient. Write the necessary information on the tape *before* you place it on the dressing.

8 Finally, label the tubing and the container, as instructed on page 43, and document the entire procedure.

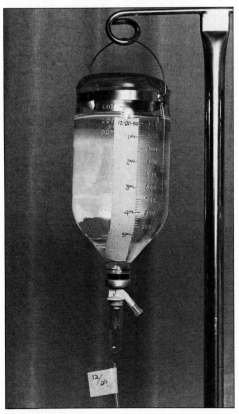

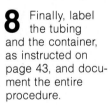

Replacing I.V. tubing

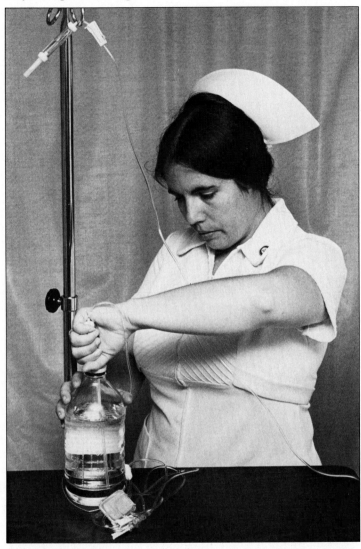

Sometimes you need to replace I.V. tubing but don't have to change the bag or bottle. Knowing what to do makes the procedure simple. Follow these steps:

Before you begin, check the dressing and site. Since you should redress the site daily, changing the tubing's often a convenient time to change the dressing too.

Now, slow the infusion to the minimum flow rate, or keep-vein-open (KVO) rate. Next, disconnect the old tubing from the bottle and either hang it on the I.V. pole hook, or tape it to the pole. Loosely cover the end of the disconnected tubing with the spike cover from the new tubing to prevent contamination. Remember, the other end's still connected to the patient, so take care to maintain sterility.

Next, clean the container's rubber stopper or port with alcohol, and spike the container with the new tubing. Flush the tubing and close the clamp. Then, carefully disconnect the old tubing and adapter, holding the needle hub with a 2" x 2" sterile gauze pad.

Now, remove the protective cap from the new tubing and quickly insert the tubing adapter into the needle or catheter hub. Readjust the flow to the prescribed rate. Relabel the tubing, as described before, and document the entire procedure.

I.V. pumps and controllers

Working with I.V. pumps

Since infusion pumps come in a wide variety of shapes, sizes, and designs, they may seem confusing to you. But the following pages will help you sort them out. We'll show you several pumps that are representative of the models available today.

Here's how they differ:
• *Syringe pump* (for example, the Auto-Syringe Syringe Pump®) compresses the syringe plunger at a controlled rate.
• *Peristaltic pump* (for example, the IVAC 530 Peristaltic Infusion Pump®) exerts pressure on the I.V. tubing, rather than the fluid itself. Most operate with ordinary I.V. tubing.
• *I.V. controller* (for example, the IVAC 230 Controller®) uses gravity to maintain a controlled flow rate. Because it doesn't exert pressure on the fluid or tubing, it's not really a pump. But, like a pump, it helps deliver fluids accurately.
• *Piston pump* (for example, the Abbott/Shaw LifeCare Pump®) controls fluid flow rate by piston action. It usually requires special tubing.

Most models can be operated by battery as well as electric current. Some compact models are portable.

🖂 *Nursing tip:* Attach a copy of the instructions to the equipment for a handy reference; then follow them carefully. Remember, a pump's accuracy depends on your skill in operating it.

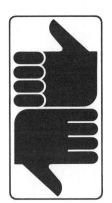

INDICATIONS/CONTRAINDICATIONS

I.V. pumps: Pros and cons

Regardless of the model, all I.V. pumps have certain advantages and disadvantages. Acquaint yourself with them before you use the equipment. This list will help.

Advantages
• They maintain a more accurate flow rate than the usual gravity and clamp system.
• They can administer a wide range of fluids, including drugs and hyperalimentation; some types even pump blood.
• They save you time because you don't need to check and readjust the flow rate constantly.
• Most types use either bags or bottles; many use ordinary I.V. tubing.
• Many can be used with in-line filters.
• Many can be used for arterial lines and nasogastric infusions.

Disadvantages
• They're complicated to operate and require some special instruction.
• They take time to set up and prime.
• They're expensive and take up storage space.
• They may create a false sense of security. Check pumps periodically to make sure they're working properly.

Using a syringe pump

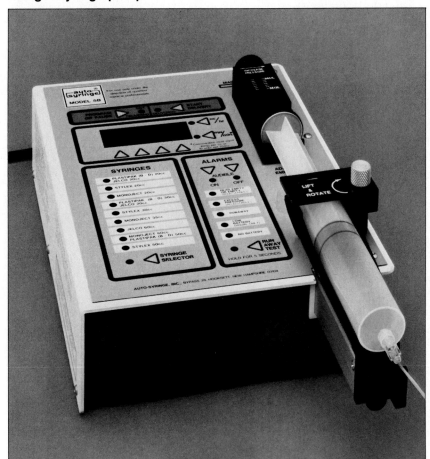

A syringe pump, like this one made by Auto-Syringe, Inc., features a disposable syringe. This syringe can deliver blood, medications, or nutrients by a variety of routes— intravenous, arterial, or subcutaneous. Because this pump can deliver small amounts of fluid very slowly (as little as .01 ml/hr), it's frequently used for infants. Its accurate low flow, or KVO rates, makes it ideal for maintaining the patency of arterial lines too. And because the syringe pump's battery-operated and portable, it's especially useful for ambulatory patients.

I.V. pumps and controllers

Using an infusion pump or controller

As you can see, the IVAC 530 Peristaltic Infusion Pump and the IVAC 230 Controller look almost the same. You can connect standard micro- or macrodrip I.V. sets to both. However, they don't work exactly the same, so before you use either, make sure you read the manufacturer's instructions carefully.

Both machines operate on a drops-per-minute rate. The peristaltic pump can infuse between 1 and 99 drops per minute; the controller infuses between 1 and 69 drops per minute. Use the conversion chart on the side of each machine to calculate milliliters-per-hour rates. Keep in mind that the I.V. container may be overfilled, either by the manufacturer or when you add medication. In such a case,

account for the overfill milliliters when you calculate the drip rate.

Neither machine can deliver more than 200 ml/hr. If you set the machine to deliver more than this, an alarm may sound.

The back panel of each features a reset button, as well as receptacles for a drop sensor attachment, external battery plugs, and a call signal.

Remember: The controller works by gravitational force, so make sure the I.V. container's located at least 30" (76 cm) above the venipuncture site. And because the controller can't exert the positive pressure of a true pump, don't use it to deliver highly viscous fluid or to keep an arterial line open.

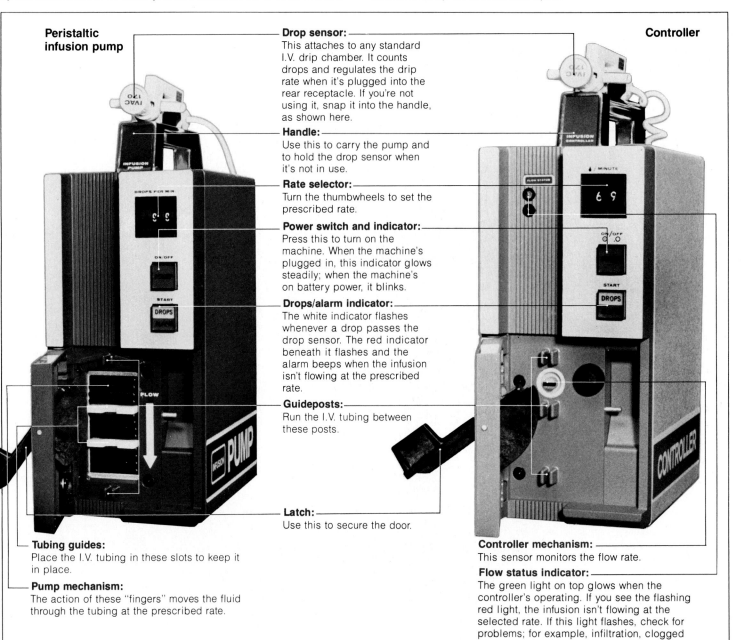

Peristaltic infusion pump

Controller

Drop sensor:
This attaches to any standard I.V. drip chamber. It counts drops and regulates the drip rate when it's plugged into the rear receptacle. If you're not using it, snap it into the handle, as shown here.

Handle:
Use this to carry the pump and to hold the drop sensor when it's not in use.

Rate selector:
Turn the thumbwheels to set the prescribed rate.

Power switch and indicator:
Press this to turn on the machine. When the machine's plugged in, this indicator glows steadily; when the machine's on battery power, it blinks.

Drops/alarm indicator:
The white indicator flashes whenever a drop passes the drop sensor. The red indicator beneath it flashes and the alarm beeps when the infusion isn't flowing at the prescribed rate.

Guideposts:
Run the I.V. tubing between these posts.

Latch:
Use this to secure the door.

Tubing guides:
Place the I.V. tubing in these slots to keep it in place.

Pump mechanism:
The action of these "fingers" moves the fluid through the tubing at the prescribed rate.

Controller mechanism:
This sensor monitors the flow rate.

Flow status indicator:
The green light on top glows when the controller's operating. If you see the flashing red light, the infusion isn't flowing at the selected rate. If this light flashes, check for problems; for example, infiltration, clogged filters, or insufficient distance between container and controller.

Setting up an infusion pump

1 *As an example of how a piston action infusion pump works, we're going to show you how to operate the Abbott/Shaw Life-Care Pump. Keep in mind that this model is a little more complicated than a peristaltic pump. Of course, no matter which model pump you use, always read the manufacturer's instructions carefully.*

Take a look at this pump's control panel. As you can see, it administers fluid in ml-per-hour, rather than drops-per-minute. In other words, it monitors the actual volume of fluid administered to the patient instead of just counting drops. As a result, accuracy is not affected by drop size, temperature, or fluid viscosity.

When the flow alarm or the dose limit alarm activates, the delivery rate is reduced to a keep-vein-open (KVO) rate of 4 ml/hr. But if the original delivery rate was less than 4 ml/hr, the lower rate will be maintained by this pump. Remember, not all pumps have this feature. Make sure the pump you're using doesn't have a KVO rate higher than the flow rate prescribed.

The pump stops delivery if the line's occluded or if infiltration's detected. (Learn about infiltration detectors on page 56.)

Piston action infusion pump

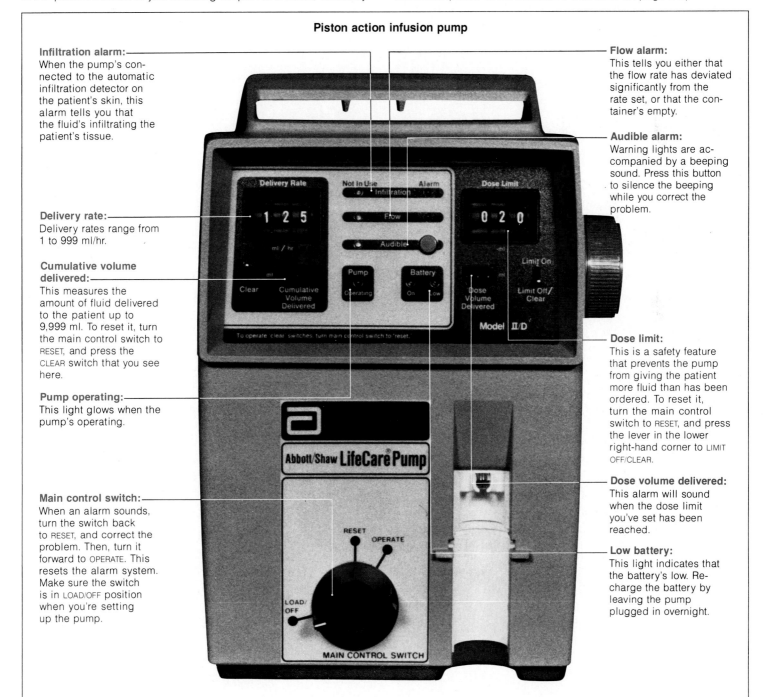

Infiltration alarm: When the pump's connected to the automatic infiltration detector on the patient's skin, this alarm tells you that the fluid's infiltrating the patient's tissue.

Delivery rate: Delivery rates range from 1 to 999 ml/hr.

Cumulative volume delivered: This measures the amount of fluid delivered to the patient up to 9,999 ml. To reset it, turn the main control switch to RESET, and press the CLEAR switch that you see here.

Pump operating: This light glows when the pump's operating.

Main control switch: When an alarm sounds, turn the switch back to RESET, and correct the problem. Then, turn it forward to OPERATE. This resets the alarm system. Make sure the switch is in LOAD/OFF position when you're setting up the pump.

Flow alarm: This tells you either that the flow rate has deviated significantly from the rate set, or that the container's empty.

Audible alarm: Warning lights are accompanied by a beeping sound. Press this button to silence the beeping while you correct the problem.

Dose limit: This is a safety feature that prevents the pump from giving the patient more fluid than has been ordered. To reset it, turn the main control switch to RESET, and press the lever in the lower right-hand corner to LIMIT OFF/CLEAR.

Dose volume delivered: This alarm will sound when the dose limit you've set has been reached.

Low battery: This light indicates that the battery's low. Recharge the battery by leaving the pump plugged in overnight.

I.V. pumps and controllers

Setting up an infusion pump continued

2 This is the tubing you'll use with the pump. As you can see, it includes two manual clamps. It also has two "Y" injection ports: one for piggybacking and one for secondary lines or I.V. push. The tubing may be either vented or nonvented, depending on the type of I.V. container you're using.

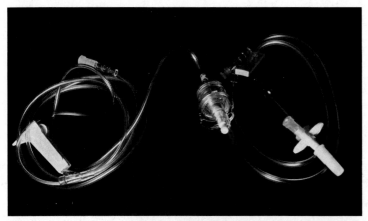

3 Now, take a closer look at the clear plastic chamber in the middle of the tubing. This is the pumping chamber, which maintains the prescribed flow rate. For the patient's safety, it's designed to trap any air that enters the tubing. The pump will automatically shut down and sound an alarm before any air reaches the patient.

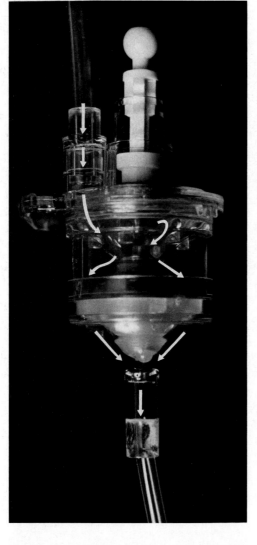

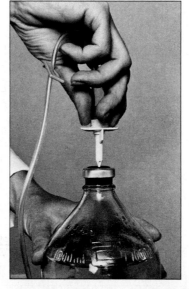

4 Now that you're acquainted with the pump's components, we'll show you how to put them together. But first, attach the pump to the I.V. pole. When you hang the I.V. container later, the pump should rest about 18" below it.

Explain the pump to your patient, and tell him about the alarm system. Let him listen to the alarm, so he won't panic if it goes off.

Get ready to spike the container and prime the tubing. But before you do, move the slide clamp 1" so it's below the drip chamber and close it, as shown in this photo. Position the flow clamp 4" to 6" below the pumping chamber and close it, too.

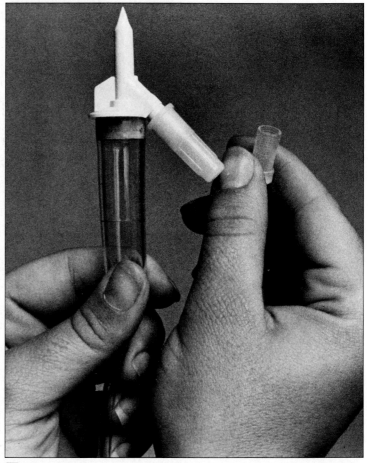

5 Then, spike and hang the I.V. container, following the same procedure explained on page 16. Don't forget to squeeze the drip chamber until it's half full. ☎ *Nursing tip:* If you're using a bag, you can convert vented tubing into nonvented tubing by removing the air filter and replacing it with the spike cover, as shown here.

6 Now you're ready to prime the pumping chamber. First, open the pumping chamber so fluid can flow through it. To do this, push in the white plunger until it locks in the down position. *Note:* Don't manipulate the plunger any more than necessary, or you may damage it.

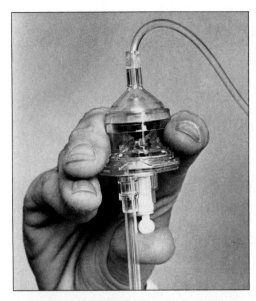

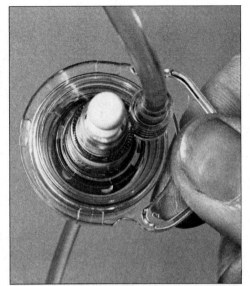

9 Close the flow clamp the moment the fluid reaches it. Then, hold the drip chamber lip, as shown here, and look down through the top for bubbles. If you see any, invert the chamber again. Open the flow clamp, and lightly tap the chamber until the bubbles disappear.

7 Open the slide clamp all the way. Use the flow clamp to set a slow flow rate. Then, invert the piggyback port, and tap it gently. *Note:* This simple step is often forgotten in the priming process. Examine the port closely and make sure no air bubbles remain trapped inside.

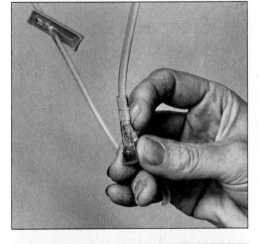

8 As the pumping chamber fills, invert it to a 45° angle, as shown in this photo. Then, quickly roll the tubing between your fingers. This wets the sides of the chamber and dispels air bubbles.

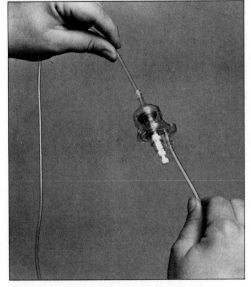

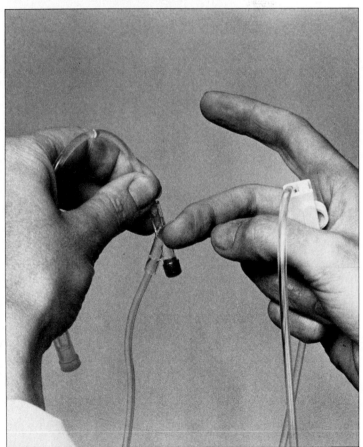

10 When you've expelled all the air from the pumping chamber, you're ready to remove all the air from the rest of the tubing. Hold the open end of the tubing over a wastebasket, and open the flow clamp all the way. As the fluid runs through, tap the secondary port to dislodge any trapped air. When the tubing's free of air, close the flow clamp again.

I.V. pumps and controllers

Setting up an infusion pump continued

11 Want to know an easier way to prime infusion pump tubing? Use this simple plastic attachment called the Abbott Accuprime adapter. After you've hung the container and filled the drip chamber to the correct level, place the adapter over the pumping chamber plunger, as shown here. Now, open both flow clamps.

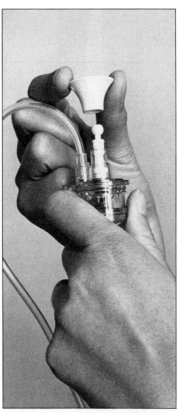

13 Now you're ready to attach the flow detector, which monitors the flow rate.
Squeeze the grip on its side, as this photo shows. Move the flow detector into position, and release the grip.

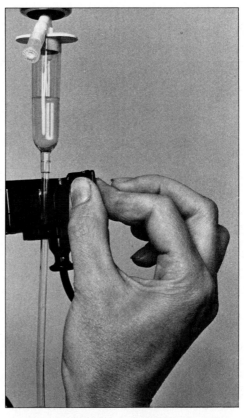

12 Next, invert the pumping chamber and adapter against a flat horizontal surface, and allow fluid to flow just past the upper Y-port. To stop the flow, lift the chamber. Clear air bubbles from the upper line.
Press the adapter against the flat surface again to fill the pumping chamber completely. Remove air bubbles in the chamber by tapping the adapter three or four times against the surface. Remove air bubbles from the lower Y-port by tapping it with your fingers.
Then, when tubing, pumping chamber, and Y-ports are all free of air, continue the procedure shown in the following photos. Don't forget to remove the Accuprime adapter before you insert the pumping chamber in the infusion pump. *Note:* Abbott supplies an Accuprime adapter with each LifeCare pump. Read the instructions thoroughly before using it.

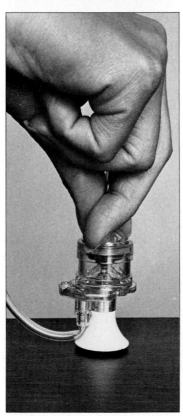

14 Or, if you prefer, just slide it into position and press firmly until it snaps into place. When the flow detector's properly in place, the edge of the grip will fit over one side of the drip chamber's lip.

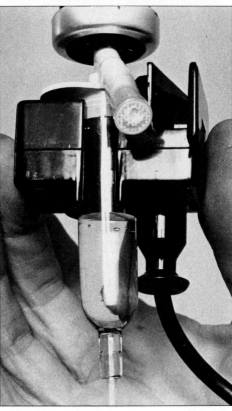

15 .Now, pull up the white plunger in the pumping chamber. This closes the pumping chamber. Of course, if you're using the Accuprime adapter, this step is unnecessary.

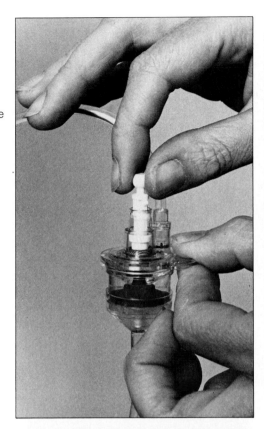

17 Set the delivery rate and the dose limit.

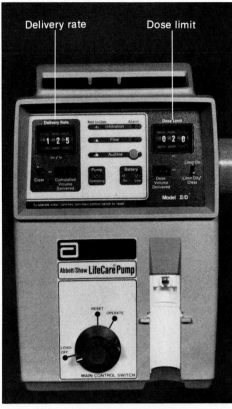

16 Turn the main control switch to the LOAD/OFF position. Hold the pumping chamber by the lip, and insert it into the slot on the front of the machine, like you see here. The chamber will lock in place.

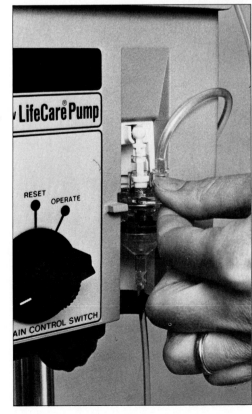

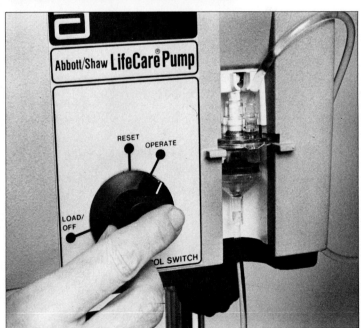

18 Finally, connect the tubing to the patient's I.V. catheter. Open the flow clamp (the slide clamp should already be open), and turn the main control switch to OPERATE.

Check your patient regularly. Don't wait for an alarm to sound before you examine him. *Remember:* The best defense against complications is an observant nurse!

I.V. pumps and controllers

Using an automatic infiltration detector

1 *This automatic infiltration detector may be used with the Abbott/Shaw LifeCare Pump. This device activates an alarm and stops the infusion if the patient's skin becomes unusually cool, which is a common sign of infiltration.*

As you can see, a large T is embossed at one end of the detector. This identifies one of the two temperature sensors in the device. The second sensor is about 1" below the T.

Here's how to use it: First, slip the infiltration detector into a sterile, disposable plastic cover, as shown here. These covers, which are available from the manufacturer, guard against contamination and let you reuse the detector.

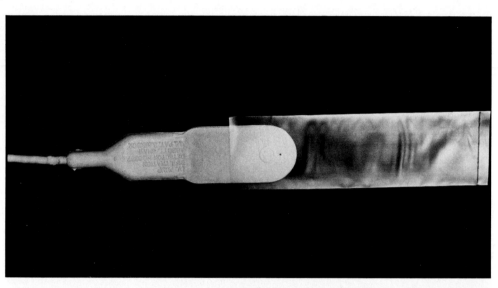

2 Now, place the detector directly on the patient's skin, positioning the *T* over the tip of the needle or catheter as it lies in the vein. Make sure the second sensor's directly against the skin too. Then, as you press each sensor firmly against the skin, secure both ends of the device with wide tape, as shown here.

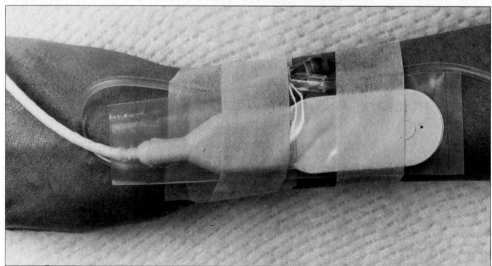

3 Fold in the corners of the plastic cover, as shown, and secure the detector cable, using the chevron method of taping. Then, plug the detector cable into the outlet at the back of the pump. Watch carefully for signs of infiltration for at least 2 minutes. (That's how long it takes the detector to start working.) *Remember:* If the prescribed flow rate is slow, the detector may not detect the early stages of infiltration. To guard against this, continue to monitor the site yourself.

Finally, check the detector periodically to make sure it's in place. Stay alert for the alarm signal which will sound if the detector buckles or pops up.

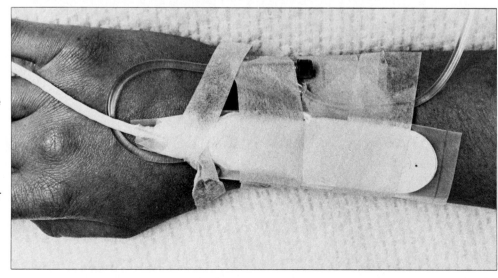

Special problems

TROUBLESHOOTING

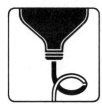

Infusion pumps: How to prevent problems

An infusion pump's only as effective as the nurse operating it. Don't expect the pump to be a substitute for your own nursing skills. You still must check the patient regularly for complications, such as infiltration or infection. (For signs and symptoms of these and other complications, see the chart on pages 58 and 59.) And the machine may not work properly all the time. Make sure you have easy access to the manufacturer's instructions and recommendations. But you can avoid several common infusion pump problems by using this checklist:

• Follow the manufacturer's instructions precisely when you insert the tubing. Remember, each model's a little different, and it's easy to make a mistake. (*Note:* To avoid overloading the patient with fluid, be sure to clamp off the tubing when the pump door's open.)

• Take care to flush *all* air out of the tubing before connecting it to the patient. The danger of air embolism increases when the fluid's under pressure.

• Double-check the flow rate. Don't assume you'll get an accurate rate just by setting the control. Monitor the flow rate yourself over a specific time span; once you determine how inaccurate the delivery rate is, you can adjust the flow accordingly.

• If your machine has a photoelectric drop sensor, position it properly. Align the top edge with the drip opening, and make sure the drip chamber's one-half to one-third full. Otherwise, the drop count won't be accurate.

• Don't let droplets cling to the sides of the drip chamber, or the drop count will be unreliable. Correct this problem by removing the drop sensor, clamping off the tubing below the chamber, and inverting the solution container and drip chamber. Repeat, if necessary. Then, replace the drop sensor, unclamp the tubing, and adjust the flow rate.

• Avoid turning the pump on and off excessively. This can clog the catheter.

• Before you attach an I.V. filter or infuse blood, check the manufacturer's recommendations. Not all pumps are designed for these purposes.

PATIENT TEACHING

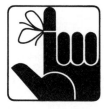

If your I.V.'s connected to an infusion pump

Dear Patient:
Your I.V. line is connected to a special pump that will keep the I.V. fluid running at the prescribed rate. Avoid touching the door latch or any of the buttons. You may disturb the setting and trigger an alarm.

If one of the alarms *does* flash or beep, don't be upset. Just call the nurse so she can correct the problem.

Suppose you're allowed to take a walk. The nurse can unplug the pump and let it operate on battery power for a short period. When she does, push the pole ahead of you, grasping the pole at pump level to keep it steady. Avoid jostling the pole as you move; otherwise, you'll set off an alarm.

Your family and friends are probably unfamiliar with the pump, too. Tell them what the pump's for so it won't make them uncomfortable.

This patient teaching aid may be reproduced by office copier for distribution to patients. ©1980, Intermed Communications, Inc.

When a child needs I.V. therapy

A child's anatomy and physiology differ significantly from an adult's. That's why the child on I.V. therapy needs your special care. First of all, a child's size makes his system less tolerant of fluid and medication overdoses. Second, a child's metabolism rate is about three times faster than an adult's. Because that rate determines the body's water requirements, a child needs much more water.

The doctor considers these factors—along with weight, size, and clinical condition—when he calculates the amount to be administered intravenously. You can help him by taking baseline readings, keeping accurate intake and output records, and watching for complications. Keep in mind that changes occur rapidly in children. Up-to-date pediatric records are essential.

You'll administer pediatric I.V. therapy with a volume-control set. Since medication doses for children are more precise, make every effort to deliver all the medication in the fluid chamber. To insure correct administration, use an infusion pump. Find out how to use one on page 50.

Remember, I.V. therapy will probably be a new and frightening procedure for the young patient. Give him all the attention and support you can. Explain the procedure in words he can understand. Answer his questions honestly. To help you, we've included a patient teaching aid designed especially for children on I.V. therapy. Look for it on page 152.

What about the parents?

An important part of pediatric care is how you deal with the parents of a child receiving I.V. therapy. The younger the child, the more he depends on his parents for support. In most cases, their moods will influence how he feels. For example, if his parents are confused and uneasy, the child may be too. So be sure to include the parents in your patient teaching sessions. Once you reassure them and they understand the procedure, they can comfort and support their child even more.

If the parents want to, let them assist you in caring for the child. Also, encourage them to stay with the child during and after therapy procedures. But don't ask them to restrain the child or help you in any way during venipuncture. When the procedure's over, remember to compliment the child on his good behavior.

Special problems

Complications from I.V. therapy

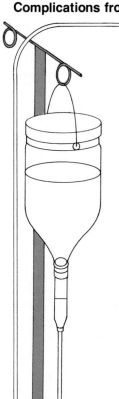

Complication	Possible causes	Signs and symptoms	Nursing considerations	Prevention tips
Infiltration	• Needle or catheter displacement (either partial or complete) • Leakage of blood around needle or catheter (especially likely in an older patient whose tissues have lost their elasticity)	• Coolness of skin around site • Swelling around site, which may or may not be painful • Swelling of entire limb • Absence of blood backflow. If a tourniquet's applied above the site, the infusion continues to run. • Sluggish flow rate	• Discontinue the infusion, and remove the needle or catheter immediately. • If the infiltration's caught within a half hour and the swelling's small, apply ice. Otherwise, apply warm wet compresses to encourage absorption. • Restart I.V. in another limb. • Document what you've done.	• Use a splint to stabilize the needle or catheter when the site's over a joint or the patient's active. • Palpate occasionally to confirm proper needle position. When a needle's placed correctly in a superficial vein, you can usually feel it easily.
Thrombophlebitis	• Injury to the vein, either during venipuncture or from needle movement later • Irritation to the vein caused by the following: long-term therapy, irritating or incompatible additives, or use of a vein that's too small to handle the amount or type of solution • Sluggish flow rate which allows a clot to form at the end of the needle or catheter	• Sluggish flow rate • Edema in limb • A vein that's sore, hard, cordlike, and warm to the touch. It may look like a red line above the venipuncture site.	• Discontinue the infusion and remove the needle or catheter immediately. • Apply warm wet compresses. • Notify doctor. • Restart I.V. in another limb. • Document what you've done. • *Important:* In the case of a sluggish flow rate, never try to irrigate the line. In addition to increasing the risk of infection, you may flush a clot into the bloodstream, causing an embolus.	• If you have to use an irritating additive, try to find a vein large enough to dilute it. Dilute irritating additives with diluents, if possible. • Make sure drug additives are compatible. • Keep the infusion flowing at the prescribed rate. • Stabilize the needle or catheter with a splint, if necessary.
Circulatory overload	• Too much fluid • Fluid delivered too fast	• Rise in blood pressure and central venous pressure (CVP) • Dilation of veins, with neck veins sometimes visibly engorged • Rapid breathing, shortness of breath, rales • Wide variance between liquid input and urine output	• Slow the infusion to a keep-vein-open (KVO) rate. • Raise patient's head. • Keep him warm to promote peripheral circulation and ease the stress on the central veins. • Monitor vital signs. • Administer oxygen, if permitted. • Notify doctor. • Document what you've done.	• Be aware of the patient's cardiovascular status and history. • Tell the doctor if the fluid volume or flow rate may be more than the patient can tolerate. • Monitor the patient's urine output.
Air embolism (Air embolisms pose a greater risk and are more common with central lines than with peripheral ones. For more details, see page 96.)	• Container allowed to run dry • Air in tubing • Loose connections	• Blood pressure drop • Rise in CVP • Weak, rapid pulse • Cyanosis • Loss of consciousness	• Turn the patient on his left side, and lower the head of the bed. If air's entered his heart chambers, this position may keep it on the right side of the heart. The pulmonary artery will then absorb small air bubbles. • Check system for leaks. • Give oxygen if allowed. • Notify doctor immediately. • Document what you've done.	• Clear all air from the tubing before attaching it to the patient. • Change containers before they're empty. • Make sure all connections are secure.

Complications from I.V. therapy continued

Complication	Possible causes	Signs and symptoms	Nursing considerations	Prevention tips
Catheter embolism (Catheter embolisms are more common with inside-the-needle catheters [INC] than with outside-the-needle catheters [ONC].)	• Withdrawing the catheter before the needle or attempting to rethread a catheter with a needle • Failure to secure the catheter to the skin adequately	• Discomfort along the vein in which the catheter fragment's lodged • Blood pressure drop • Rise in CVP • Weak, rapid pulse • Cyanosis • Loss of consciousness	• Discontinue I.V. • Apply tourniquet above site. You may be able to stop the catheter from migrating farther. • Have patient X-rayed to confirm embolism. • Document what you've done.	• Remember to withdraw needle and catheter together after an unsuccessful venipuncture attempt. • Take special care when taping or withdrawing an INC.
Infection of venipuncture site	• Poor aseptic techniques; for example, failure to keep the site clean or to change I.V. equipment regularly	• Swelling and soreness at site • Foul-smelling discharge	• Discontinue infusion, and remove needle or catheter immediately. Send I.V. equipment to the lab for bacterial analysis. • Culture drainage. • Clean site, apply antimicrobial ointment, and cover with sterile gauze pad. • Restart I.V. in another limb. • Document what you've done.	• Review and improve aseptic technique. • *Remember:* Wash your hands thoroughly before beginning any I.V. procedure.
Systemic infection (more common with plastic catheters than with metal needles)	• Poor aseptic technique • Contamination of equipment during manufacture, storage, or use • Irrigation of clogged I.V.	• Sudden rise in temperature and pulse • Chills and shaking • Blood pressure changes	• Look for other sources of infection first. Culture urine, sputum, and blood, as ordered. • Discontinue the I.V. immediately, and send all I.V. equipment to the lab for bacterial analysis. • Restart I.V. in another limb. • Notify doctor. • Document what you've done.	• Review and improve aseptic technique. • Take care not to contaminate the site when bathing the patient. • If any part of the system's accidentally disconnected, don't rejoin it. Instead, replace the parts with sterile equipment.
Speed shock	• Drugs administered too quickly • Improper administration of bolus infusions	• Flushed face • Headache • Tight feeling in chest • Irregular pulse • Loss of consciousness • Shock • Cardiac arrest	• Discontinue drug infusion. • Begin an infusion of 5% dextrose in water at KVO rate. You must keep the vein open for emergency treatment. • Notify doctor immediately. • Document what you've done.	• Keep infusion flowing at prescribed rate.
Allergic reaction	• Sensitivity to an I.V. fluid (especially an additive)	• Itching • Rash • Shortness of breath	• Slow infusion to KVO rate. • Notify doctor. • Document what you've done.	• Ask the patient if he has any allergies before beginning venipuncture procedures. Remember, he may have a sensitivity to iodine used as a skin prep.

Special problems

PATIENT TEACHING

Helping the ambulatory patient

When an ambulatory patient's undergoing I.V. therapy, she'll need special care to keep her infusion flowing properly. To provide her with that care, follow these guidelines:
• Position the pole to allow 30" to 36" between the venipuncture site and the container. *Remember:* The flow rate's affected whenever the distance between container and needle changes. So, don't forget to readjust the height of the pole when she sits in a chair.
• Instruct the patient to keep the venipuncture site below her heart. Tell her to use her other arm for routine tasks.
• Watch for any changes in flow rate. Sometimes an active patient jostles the flow clamp open. Tell her to notify a nurse if she notices any difference in the flow rate. Warn her not to tamper with the flow clamp herself.
• Teach your patient how to move the I.V. pole. Your advice will vary from patient to patient; for example, it'll depend on how active she is, where the needle's positioned, and how much tubing's involved. Use your common sense. Try to arrange things so that the tubing won't tangle in front of her or get caught in the pole's wheels.
Nursing tip: For safety's sake, remove the bedside table and other unnecessary equipment from the side of the bed nearest her venipuncture site. Keep only the I.V. pole and the patient's slippers on that side so she'll have them within reach.

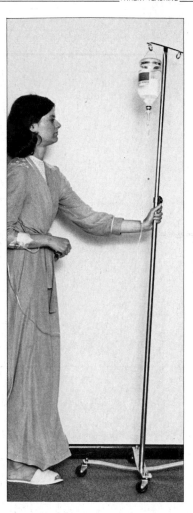

When the patient's on bed rest: Helpful tips

Whether or not your patient's ambulatory, you'll try to position her I.V. equipment so she'll be comfortable and safe. But when she's on bed rest, you may find these additional guidelines helpful:
• Attach the patient's I.V. pole to the bed, so the distance between the venipuncture site and the solution container doesn't change when the bed's raised or lowered.
• If the patient's restless, extension tubing will give her more freedom without straining the line.
• Tell her not to kink or compress the tubing as she moves, and remind her not to tamper with it. Otherwise, she may dislodge the needle or catheter, or even pull the spike out of the container.

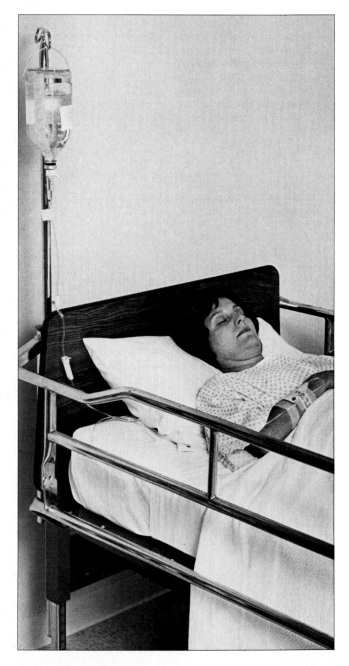

Your I.V.: What you should know

Dear Patient:
You're receiving intravenous (I.V.) therapy so the fluid or medicine your body needs can flow directly into your veins. Once the I.V.'s in place, you'll feel no discomfort and will probably be able to move around with few restrictions. But remember to keep the arm the I.V.'s attached to at waist level, and use your other arm for routine tasks.

If, at any time during your therapy, you have any questions about the I.V. equipment or dressing, call the nurse. For example, let her know if you notice:
• Burning, pain, swelling, or redness near the point of needle insertion
• Blood backed up in the tubing
• I.V. fluid running very quickly through the tubing (or not running at all)
• Wetness around the dressing or along the tubing
• Loose tape on the dressing.

This patient teaching aid may be reproduced by office copier for distribution to patients.
© 1980, Intermed Communications, Inc.

TROUBLESHOOTING

Correcting obvious flow rate problems

When your patient's infusion is running too slowly, or not at all, the problem may be easily corrected. Begin by looking for the obvious. Then check to see if:
• the container's empty. If it is, replace it.
• the drip chamber's less than half full. Squeeze it until the fluid reaches the proper level.
• the flow clamp's closed. Readjust it to restore the proper drip rate.
• the tubing's kinked or caught under the patient. Untangle the line or reposition the patient.

• the container's less than 3' (1 m) above the site. Readjust the height of the I.V. pole.
• the tubing's dangling below the site and gravity's preventing the solution from reaching the patient. To remedy this problem, replace the tubing with a shorter piece, or tape some of the excess tubing to the I.V. pole (just below the flow clamp). If you tape the tubing, make sure you don't kink it accidentally.
• an air bubble's in the tubing. Tap the tubing until the bubble rises into the container.

Correcting other flow rate problems

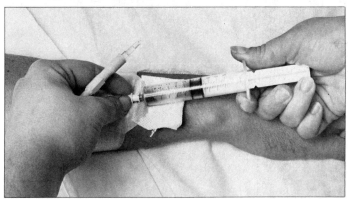

1 *Suppose your patient's I.V. isn't running at the prescribed rate and you've already looked for obvious problems. Do you know what to do next? Consider these possibilities.*

Sometimes a clot in the needle or catheter blocks the infusion. Close the flow clamp, and try aspirating the clot with a syringe on the catheter hub. (Take care not to contaminate the hub or the tubing.) If that doesn't work, restart the I.V. in another vein. *Important:* Never try irrigating a clogged I.V. with a syringe and solution. You'll increase the chance of infection and risk propelling the clot into the bloodstream.

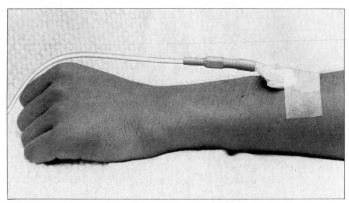

3 In some cases, you can restore flow by changing the angle of the needle or catheter. To do this, elevate it slightly with a sterile cotton ball, a 2" x 2" gauze pad, or a tongue blade. In this photo, we've left the catheter and tubing untaped for clarity, but you should secure them properly. *Note:* Never tape so tightly that blood flow's impeded.

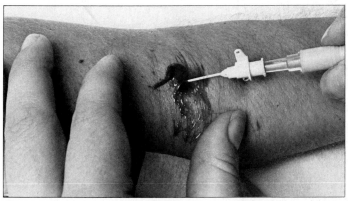

2 If the infusion's running sluggishly, the needle or catheter may be jammed against the vein wall. Try pulling it back slightly (about ⅛"). You may also try rotating a catheter gently, but don't manipulate a winged-tip needle this way. If you do, the needle's bevel may injure the vein, triggering infiltration or thrombophlebitis.

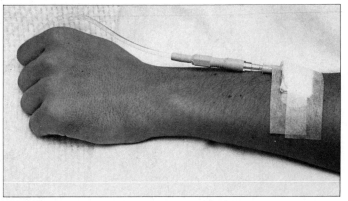

4 To lower a catheter slightly, put a sterile cotton ball, a 2" x 2" gauze pad, or a tongue blade over it, and secure it with tape. *Remember:* The needle or catheter angle may be affected by patient movement. If you find the drip rate varies when the patient moves his arm, apply a splint to stabilize the needle or catheter.

Special problems

Correcting other flow rate problems continued

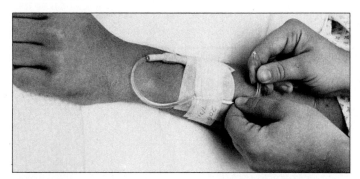

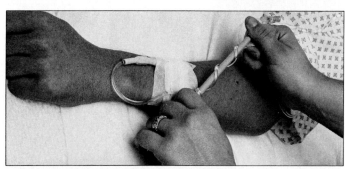

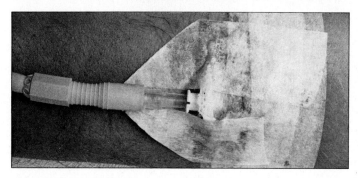

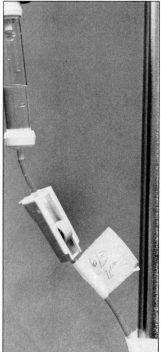

5 Here's another way to revive a sluggish I.V.: First, pinch the tubing near the site. If the line includes a flashbulb, compress it once or twice. If it doesn't have a flashbulb, compress the tubing between your fingers or with the side of a pencil. Gently squeeze about 6" to 8" of the tubing closest to the site.

6 Or, you may prefer to use this alternative: Pinch the tubing, and wrap it around a pencil four or five times. Then, quickly pull the pencil out of the tubing coil you've made.

7 Occasionally, you may discover that the infusion's running too quickly. Look first for a soaked dressing. This usually means that the needle or catheter has worked out of the skin underneath the dressing. If so, restart the I.V. in another vein.

8 If the needle or catheter seems secure, check the flow clamp. Sometimes an active patient stretches the tubing, which damages the flow clamp's effectiveness. If this happens, replace the tubing with a longer line. As an added precaution, tape the tubing to the I.V. pole to protect the clamp from stress, as shown here.

How to discontinue an I.V.

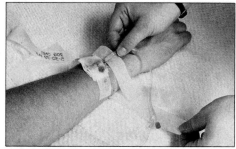

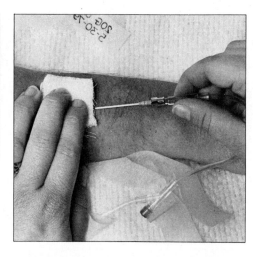

1 First, wash your hands thoroughly. Then, stop the patient's I.V. fluid flow completely by closing off the flow clamp. Carefully untape and remove the dressing, taking care not to disturb the needle or catheter.

2 Hold a 2" x 2" sterile gauze pad just above the site. Then, quickly withdraw the needle or catheter, pulling straight back to avoid tearing the vein. Immediately apply pressure to the site with a 2" x 2" sterile gauze pad, and hold it against the site until the bleeding's stopped. This prevents blood from oozing out of the vein and causing a hematoma. Finally, tape down the pad, and leave it in place for 10 minutes. Don't use an adhesive bandage strip, because it won't exert enough pressure to stop the bleeding. And don't apply alcohol; it will irritate the wound and inhibit clotting.

I.V. admixtures

What do you do for the patient who needs the slow, continuous infusion of a medication that can be diluted? Prepare an admixture by adding medication directly to a primary I.V. solution. Test your knowledge of admixtures with these questions:

What's the greatest hazard in admixture use? When's an admixture indicated and when isn't it? What's the correct technique for preparing an admixture? Not sure of your answers? Read the next few pages carefully. You'll learn everything you need to know about admixtures.

Assembling equipment

Before you prepare any admixtures for I.V. therapy, make sure your equipment's sterile and in working order, and that your medication's not outdated. Gather together what's pictured in this photo.

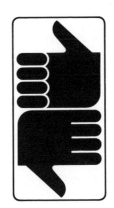

___INDICATIONS/CONTRAINDICATIONS___

When to use admixtures

As you know, admixtures are a common and widely used type of I.V. therapy.

You'll give it to patients who need:
• fluid and electrolyte maintenance and replacement; for example, KCl
• slow, continuous drug administration for diagnostic or therapeutic use; for example, Solu-B and C.

Avoid using admixtures for patients who require:
• rapid drug administration
• intermittent administration of fluids and electrolytes
• drugs that are insoluble in water or incompatible with the solution; for example, phenytoin.

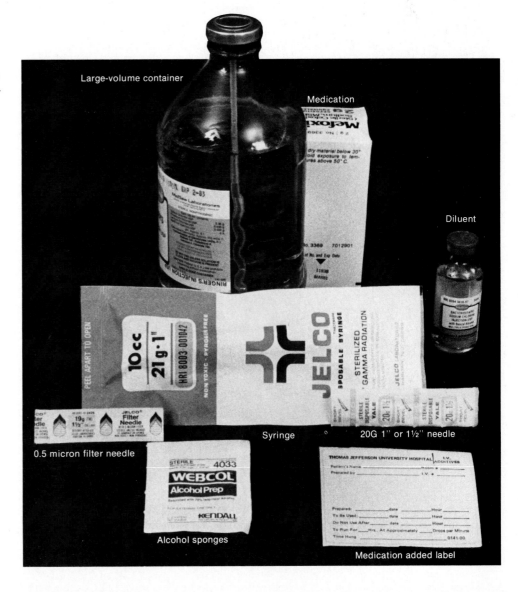

Large-volume container

Medication

Diluent

10cc 21g·1"

0.5 micron filter needle

JELCO

Syringe

20G 1" or 1½" needle

WEBCOL Alcohol Prep

Alcohol sponges

Medication added label

I.V. admixtures

Preventing incompatibility and instability

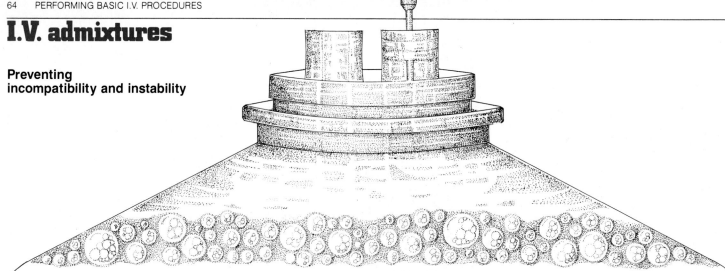

An incompatibility is an undesired physio-chemical reaction between a drug and a primary container, a primary solution, or another drug. The action destroys the drug's therapeutic effect or creates new and unwanted ones. You can prevent this type of reaction by knowing about the drugs and solutions you're mixing.

Stability refers to how long a drug retains, within specified limits, the same properties and characteristics it possessed when manufactured. The limit on stability for all drugs has been set at 10% by the United States government. So when a drug is said to be stable, at least 90% of its properties are effective until a specific date. If it loses more than 10% of its effectiveness, it's considered unstable. The general term incompatibility, in practical usage, refers to instability as well.

Types of incompatibilities
• Physical: Most physical incompatibilities result from inadequate solubility and from acid/base reactions. A physical incompatibility has occurred when you see precipitation, color change, gas release, or cloudiness in the bottle. For example, when diazepam is mixed with 5% dextrose in water, the solution becomes cloudy.
• Chemical: A chemical incompatibility, which may not always be visible, is the irreversible breakdown of a drug, producing therapeutically inactive or toxic products. For example, mixing carbenicillin disodium with gentamicin sulfate deactivates the gentamicin. Some chemical instabilities can't be prevented. Take, for example, hydrolysis and oxidation.

Hydrolysis most commonly occurs in hyperalimentation solutions and fat emulsions. This reaction produces substances that may be more acidic than the original drug, may discolor the solution, and may be toxic or sensitizing. Hydrolysis doesn't

necessarily alter the drug's therapeutic effect.

Oxidation occurs when the drug or solution experiences electron or hydrogen loss, or an oxygen increase. It causes the drug or solution to turn pink, red, or brown and makes it therapeutically ineffective.

Four factors affect compatibility
• Concentration of the drug—the stronger the drug's concentration, the swifter it may become incompatible or unstable.
• Length of contact time—the longer the drugs are in contact (either because they're prepared before they're needed or because of long administration time), the greater the chance that the mixture will become incompatible or unstable.
• Ionic strength of the drug—the lesser the drug's ionic strength, the greater the chance of incompatibility or instability.
• pH level of the mixture—when a drug's added to a primary solution, the solution's pH may be altered considerably. Many drugs, especially antibiotics, are unstable in alkaline (pH above 8) or in acidic (pH below 4) solutions. Some solutions, such as fructose, decompose if they're made alkaline by the addition of a drug like calcium, which causes the pH to exceed 7. This admixture is considered incompatible.

What buffers do
Buffers are substances added to drugs or solutions during manufacture to maintain a desired pH. Although drugs often have their own buffer, it's usually too weak to counteract the pH change that occurs when the drug's added to a strongly acidic or alkaline I.V. solution. This change in pH can cause the drug to separate from the primary solution. Potassium penicillin G, for example, is considered most stable in the pH range of 6 to 7. But if you add it to a 5% dextrose in water solution, along with other

highly buffered drugs that make the solution alkaline (amphotericin B or cephalothin solution), potassium penicillin G rapidly deteriorates. The ideal pH for I.V. fluids is approximately 7.4, the pH of blood.

General precautions when preparing I.V. admixtures
• Add one drug at a time to the primary I.V. solution. Mix and examine it thoroughly before adding the next drug.
• Add the most concentrated or most soluble drug to the solution first, since some incompatibilities, such as precipitates, require a certain concentration or amount of time to develop. Mix it well, and then add the dilute drugs.
• Remember that chemical analogues or families of drugs react similarly, though not necessarily identically. If one drug in a class is incompatible with the desired solution, other drugs in that class may be incompatible too.
• You'll find some precipitates are too fine or too clear to detect visually. Using colored additives may make it even harder. You should add additives such as riboflavin in vitamin B complex (yellow color) to the solution last to avoid masking possible precipitates or cloudiness.
• Even though contact time has been shortened with the use of minicontainers and backcheck valves, you must always check for compatibility and stability.
• If you don't have a clear understanding of the compatibility or stability of the admixtures you're using, check the manufacturer's recommendations, and consult with a pharmacist.
• Because of the complexity of this subject, many hospitals allow only registered pharmacists to prepare admixtures. But if this isn't your hospital's policy, make sure, before you begin, to have several drug references handy.

Administering admixtures

1 *How do you prepare and administer an I.V. admixture? If it's premixed or available as a liquid, you can add it directly to the I.V. solution container. However, if it's a powder, you'll have to reconstitute it. To find out how, see page 67.*

Begin the admixture procedure by swabbing the top of the medication vial. Then, use a filter needle and syringe to draw up the correct amount of medication.

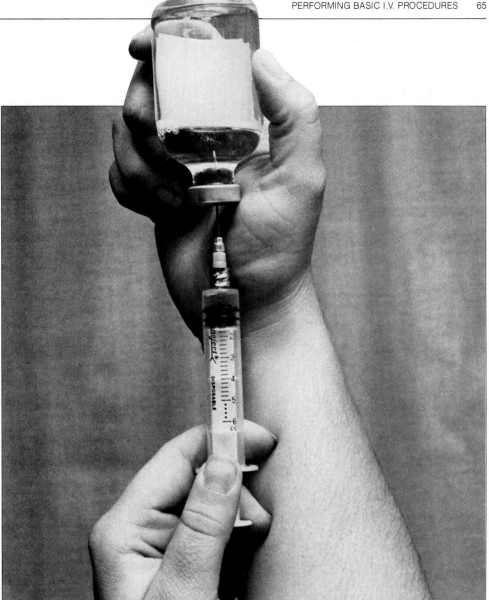

2 Replace the filter needle with a regular 1½" large-bore needle. *Remember:* A filter needle's good only once. If you force the medication back through it, you'll contaminate the medication and will have to start over. Leave the cap on the needle to minimize the risk of contamination.

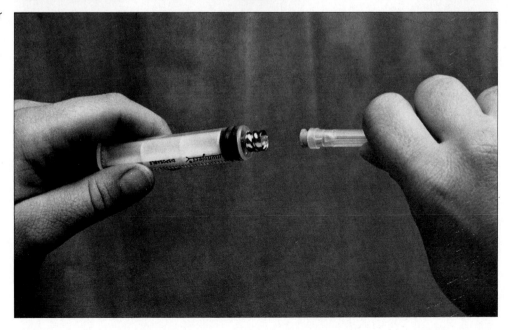

I.V. admixtures

Administering admixtures continued

3 Remove the cap from the top of the primary I.V. solution container. Swab the port with alcohol.

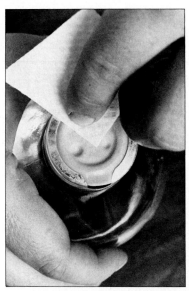

4 Uncap the medication syringe. Insert it into the port, and inject the medication. *Note:* If you're not using the primary solution immediately, cover it with a sterile additive cap available from the manufacturer.

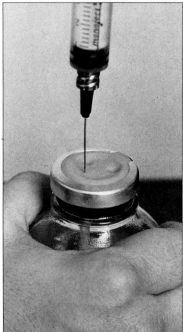

5 Gently rotate the container to mix the solution. Remember to add a timing label and a label noting the added medication, time, date, your initials.

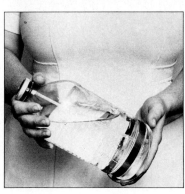

6 Spike and hang the container, following the procedure explained on page 16.

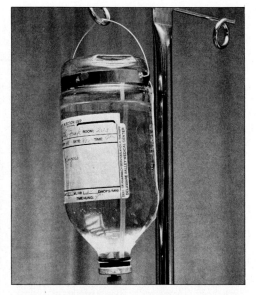

7 Then, perform venipuncture, using the same method shown earlier. When you finish, document the entire procedure.

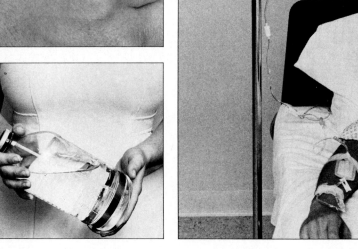

Reconstituting medication

1 *If the medication you're using comes in powder form, you must reconstitute it before delivering it. To do so, follow these steps:* Remove the protective cap from the diluent container. Swab the stopper with alcohol, as shown in this photo.

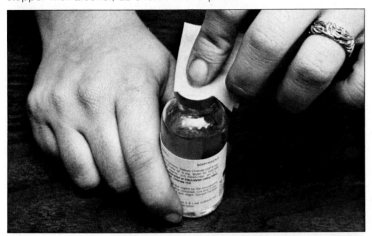

2 Draw up the recommended amount of diluent with a large-bore (18G) needle and syringe.

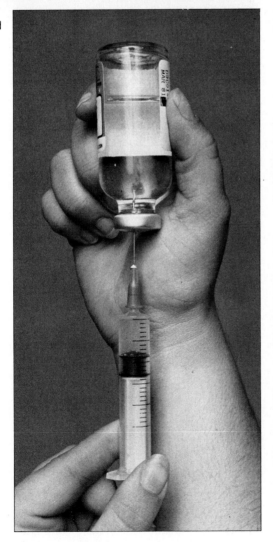

3 Swab the stopper of the drug vial with alcohol. Then, inject the diluent into the vial.

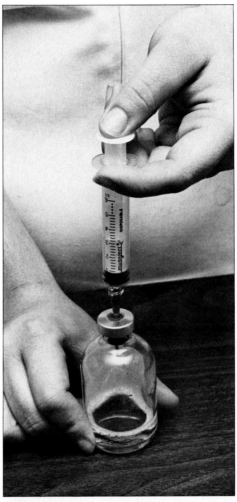

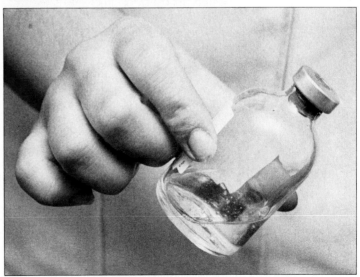

4 Mix the drug and diluent as directed. You'll know it's completely reconstituted when you can't see any particles or bubbles in the solution.

I.V. admixtures

Using a double-headed pin

1 *If you want an easy way to transfer a solution into a vacuum-sealed bottle, use a double-headed pin. A double-headed pin has two needles mounted back to back on a cap or stopper. It's encased in a plastic cover to prevent contamination.*

This photostory shows a nurse using the double-headed pin to add lidocaine to an I.V. solution. However, you can apply these steps to any double-headed pin procedure.

Here's what to do: First, remove the medication bottle's metal collar, and swab the stopper with alcohol.

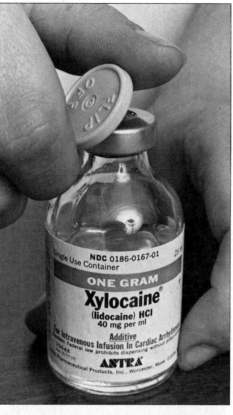

2 Leaving the plastic cover intact, insert one of the needles through the stopper. Then remove the cover.

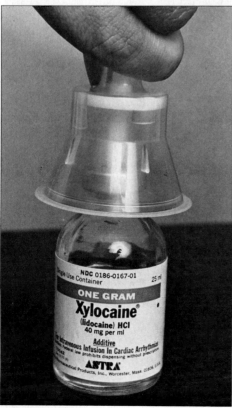

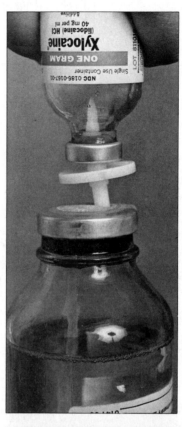

3 Now, pull the metal collar off the primary solution (or diluent) bottle, and swab the stopper or rubber diaphragm underneath. Puncture the stopper or diaphragm with the other needle. The vacuum in the primary solution bottle will pull the medication through the needles.

Important: Make sure you puncture the vacuum-sealed bottle last, so the vacuum's not lost. However, if both bottles are vacuum sealed, the order in which you puncture them isn't important.

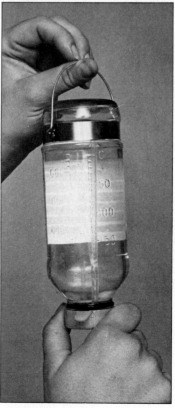

4 Follow the recommended mixing procedure. If you do it correctly, you won't see any foam or particles in the solution before you administer it.

Using an ampule transfer device

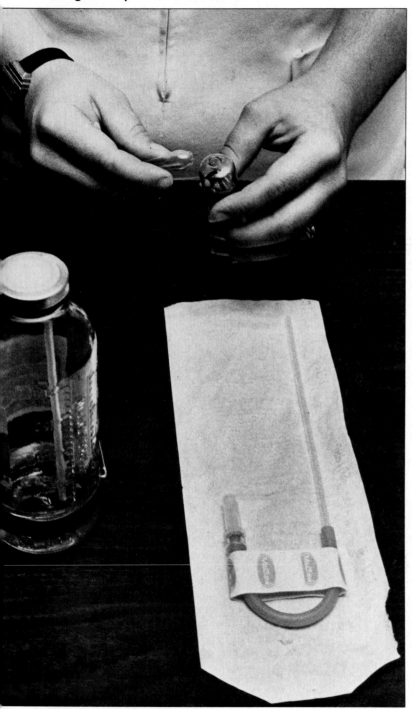

1 *Using a transfer device, like this one made by McGaw Laboratories, makes it easy to transfer fluid from an ampule to an I.V. bottle. You'll find it's more effective than a filter needle, because the filter's built right into the transfer device, reducing the chance for touch contamination. Here's how it works:*

First, remove the protective cap from the I.V. bottle, and swab the stopper with alcohol. With a fresh swab, clean the ampule neck. Then, grasp the neck and break off the top of the ampule. If you wish, protect your hands with a 4" x 4" sterile gauze pad.

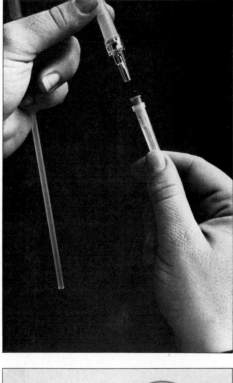

2 Next, take the transfer device out of it's wrapper. Open the package according to the manufacturer's directions. Then, remove the protective cap from the larger end of the device, and attach a needle (18G or smaller). To avoid contaminating either end of the transfer device, hold it as shown in this photo.

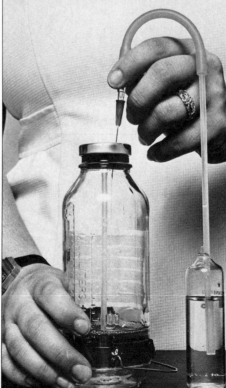

3 Now, push the open end of the transfer device all the way into the ampule. Holding the transfer device firmly, puncture the I.V. bottle stopper with the needle. The bottle's vacuum will pull fluid from the ampule into the bottle. As the fluid level in the ampule drops, tilt the ampule to keep the tip of the transfer device submerged.

I.V. admixtures

How to add medications to three types of hanging containers

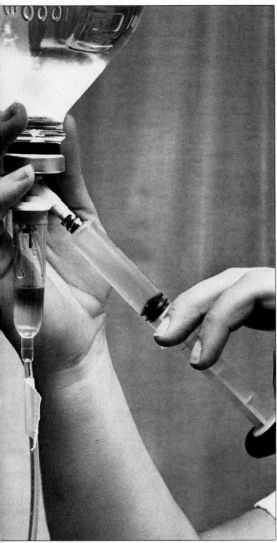

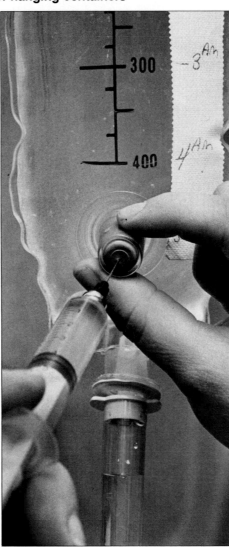

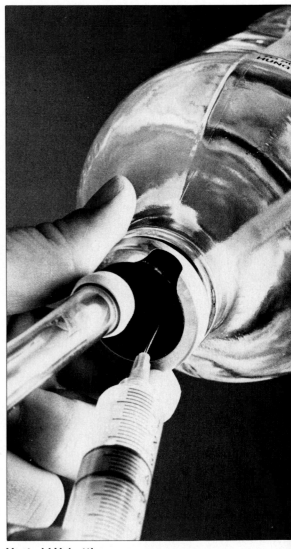

I.V. bottle with vented tubing

Suppose your I.V. set has a bottle with vented tubing. And after it's hanging, you want to add medication to the solution. First, remove the needle from the medication syringe. Then, close the flow clamp. Stopping the flow is an important step in this procedure. If you forget to do it, you could mainline the drug, creating a medication bolus, and endanger the patient's life. Next, detach the air vent from the primary I.V. tubing, making sure you don't touch the ends and contaminate them. Then, as this photo shows, insert the syringe into the air vent port, and inject the medication. Now, replace the air vent, and gently rotate the container to mix the solution. Finally, open the flow clamp, and adjust the flow rate. Label the bottle with the added medication, time and date of addition, and your initials. Document the procedure.

I.V. bag

How do you add medication to an I.V. bag that's already hanging? Before you begin, make sure there's enough solution in the bag for proper dilution. Then, close the flow clamp to avoid giving your patient a medication bolus. Next, swab the medication port with alcohol, and inject the medication into the bag. Gently rotate the bag to mix the solution. Attach a medication added label to the bag. Finally, open the clamp, and adjust the rate. Document what you've done.

Vented I.V. bottle

If you must add medication to an I.V. bottle with an indwelling vent, here's what to do: First, close the flow clamp. Don't forget to do it; if you neglect this important step, you may cause your patient to have a medication bolus.

Next, examine the stopper on the inverted bottle. You'll see a triangle imprinted on it. Swab the triangle with alcohol. Insert the medication syringe needle through the triangle, and inject the medication. Gently rotate the bottle to mix the medication with the I.V. solution. Finally, open the flow clamp, and adjust the flow rate. Label the bottle, and document what you've done.

Additive sets

At some time you'll have to administer medication by special procedure to the I.V. therapy patient. What if the drug can't be mixed with the primary solution? What if you must give it slowly or intermittently? What if it's a combination of these considerations? In such cases, you'll use an additive set.

Will you know which additive method to choose? Which procedure's correct? What complications may arise? If you're not sure, read the following pages. They'll tell you all about additive sets.

Defining additive set terms

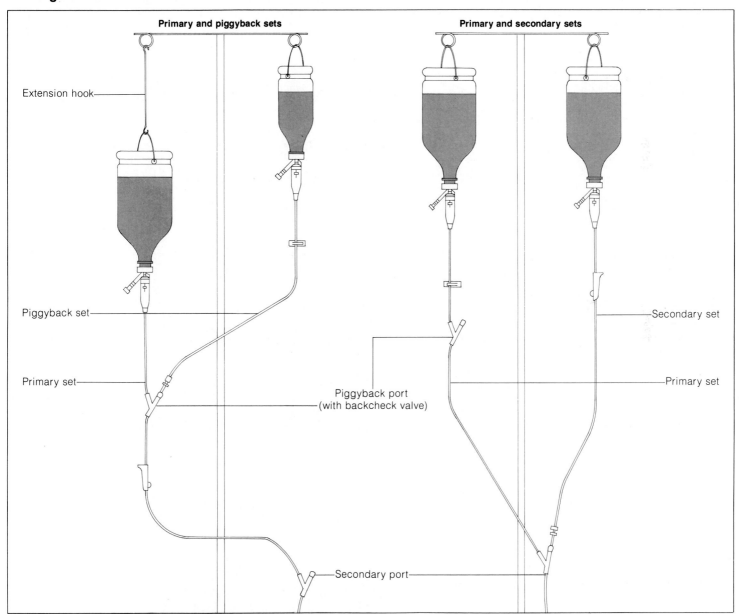

Primary and piggyback sets

Extension hook

Piggyback set

Primary set

Piggyback port
(with backcheck valve)

Secondary port

Primary and secondary sets

Secondary set

Primary set

Piggyback and secondary. How can you tell them apart? These two terms are so confusing that we can't begin to talk about additive sets until we've clarified them.

A piggyback set, shown on the left, includes a small I.V. bottle, short tubing, and usually a macrodrip system. This set connects into a primary line's upper Y-port, also called the piggyback port. A piggyback set is used solely for intermittent drug administration. For the set to work, you must position the primary I.V. container below the piggyback container. An extension hook's provided by the manufacturer for that purpose.

A secondary set, shown on the right, features an I.V. bottle (any size), long tubing, and either a microdrip or a macrodrip system. The set connects into the primary line's lower Y-port, which is also called the secondary port. As you probably know, a secondary set's used to administer drugs intermittently *or* simultaneously with a primary solution.

Additive sets

INDICATIONS/CONTRAINDICATIONS

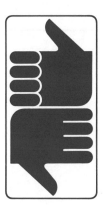

Using additive sets

When a patient with a primary I.V. line also requires intermittent administration of medication, use an I.V. additive set. It will enable you to:
• Maintain peak drug levels in the patient's bloodstream
• Avoid irritation from I.V. bolus
• Administer different drugs at different times.

Two of the most common drugs administered in this way are aminophylline and Keflin.

However, never use an I.V. additive set when the drug you're giving must be given slowly or well diluted; for example, vitamins or KCl.

PATIENT PREPARATION

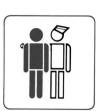

When you're using an additive set: Caring for your patient

Before you begin using an additive set, explain to the patient why you're hanging another bottle. Tell him how it works, and answer his questions honestly. By doing so, you can help minimize his fears and make him more comfortable.

Stay alert for signs of drug sensitivity in your patient, especially after the first dose. To read his reaction accurately, you'll need reference points. Establish them by getting the answers to these questions before you start:
• What are his known allergies?
• Does he have a skin condition (like hives) that'll make drug sensitivity difficult to assess?
• Is he uncomfortable or experiencing chills?
• What's his urine output?
• What's his temperature, pulse, respiratory rate, and blood pressure?

If his condition seems to contraindicate the drug, check with the doctor before you deliver it.

During administration, watch the patient closely for signs of drug sensitivity. If he shows any, discontinue delivery immediately and call a doctor. When you complete administration, assess the patient's condition again. Because you've established reference points, you can accurately judge how the drug's affected him.

Assembling equipment

Before you begin any procedure requiring an I.V. additive set, assemble all the equipment you'll need. Make sure each piece is sterile and in good working order. The first photo features equipment used in every additive set procedure. The three photos beneath it feature all the equipment you'll need for special procedures.

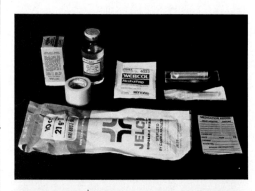

• Medication
• Syringe
• Large-bore (18G) needle
• Filter needle
• Medication added label
• Diluent
• Alcohol swab
• Adhesive tape

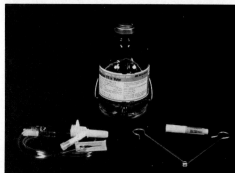

The partial-fill additive set procedure also requires:
• Minibottle
• Macrodrip tubing
• 20G 1" needle
• Extension hook

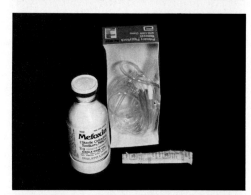

The manufacturer's secondary set procedure also requires:
• Manufacturer's drug vial
• Tubing
• 20G 1" needle
• Double-headed pin (optional)
See step 4 on the next page for details.

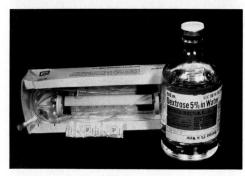

The volume-control set procedure also requires:
• 20G 1" needle
• Volume-control tubing
• 5% dextrose in water

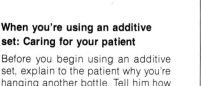

Setting up a secondary line

1 *Here's the general procedure for establishing a secondary line. To illustrate it, we're using a 250 ml bottle of medication.* Begin by reading the medication package insert. If you need to reconstitute the medication, follow the steps on page 67. Then, draw up the medication with a filter needle and syringe. Remember, a filter needle's good only once. Replace it immediately with a large-bore (18G) 1½" needle.

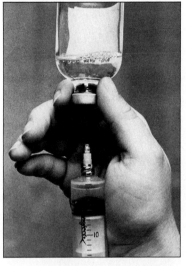

2 Swab the secondary bottle stopper with alcohol. Then, inject the medication into the secondary bottle. Gently rotate it to mix the solution.

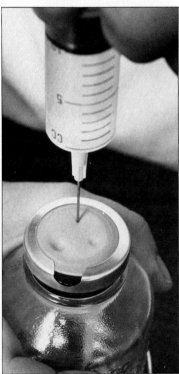

3 Affix a *medication added* label to the container. Include drug dose; date and time; expiration date (if pertinent); patient's name, and room and bed number. Remember to initial it.

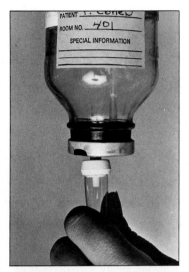

4 Attach the tubing to the secondary bottle by driving the spike into the bottle stopper. Hang the set.
   Note: Some medications now come in vials suitable for hanging directly on an I.V. pole. With this type, you don't have to prepare medication and inject it into a bottle. Instead, you can inject diluent directly into the medication vial. Then, spike the vial, prime the tubing, and hang the set as usual.

5 Attach a 20G 1" needle to the tubing adapter. Prime the entire secondary set.
   Make sure the medication's compatible with the primary line solution. If it *isn't,* swab the secondary port. Then, flush the primary tubing with saline solution before inserting the set's needle.

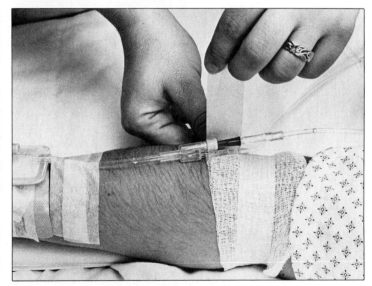

6 If the medication *is* compatible, simply swab the secondary port and insert the 20G 1" needle. Use two 3" strips of ¼" tape to secure the needle in the port, as shown here.
   Begin infusing the medication at the prescribed rate. Follow the doctor's orders; he may want it to run with the primary solution, or he may want it to run by itself. Document what you've done.

Additive sets

How to use a partial-fill piggyback set

1 *Does your patient need the intermittent infusion of a diluted drug? Then use a partial-fill piggyback set to deliver it. Here's how:* Begin the partial-fill piggyback procedure by following the steps for adding medication to a primary I.V. line. Swab the container. Read the medication's directions. If it needs to be reconstituted, turn to page 67 to find out how. If it's ready for use, draw the medication into a syringe. Then, insert the needle into the partial-fill piggyback, and inject the medication.

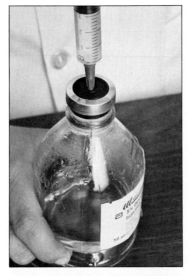

2 Label the piggyback bottle with the following information: the medication added, the date and time of addition, and your initials. Be sure you invert the label so it's right side up when the bottle's hung.

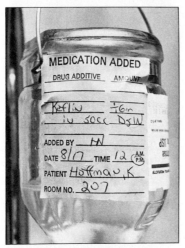

3 Now, close the piggyback line flow clamp. Push the spike into the top of the piggyback bottle, as shown here.

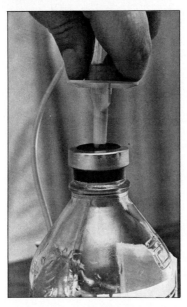

4 Turn your attention to the needle. Usually the needle's included in the piggyback set. But if it's not, attach an 18G or 19G 1" needle to the line. Don't use a needle over 1" long because it'll puncture the tubing. Open the flow clamp for a few seconds to prime the tubing and needle. Then close it again.

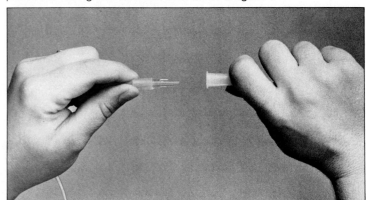

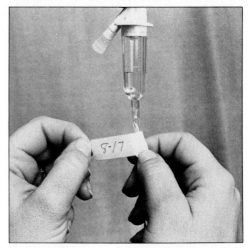

5 Label the secondary tubing with the date and time you establish the line. *Remember:* You should replace piggyback tubing every 48 hours, as recommended by the Center for Disease Control. Hang the set on the remaining I.V. pole hook.

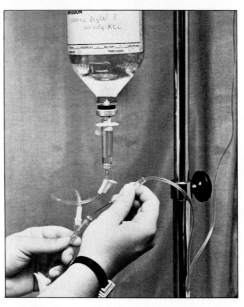

6 Swab the piggyback port of the primary I.V. line with alcohol. Make sure the medication you're administering is compatible with the primary I.V. solution. If it's not, you must flush the primary I.V. line with saline solution before connecting the piggyback line. If it is compatible, insert the piggyback set needle into the port, as shown here. Tape it securely.

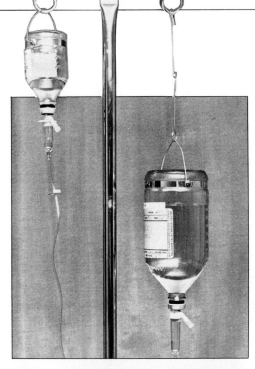

7 Use the extension hook provided to rehang the primary container. Its center of gravity must be lower than the minibottle.

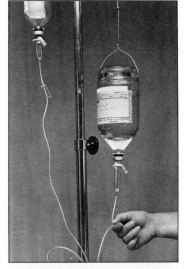

9 When the piggyback solution level drops below the drip chamber of the primary container, the backcheck valve cuts off the *piggyback* flow. Then, the primary solution automatically begins running again.

Note: Suppose you want to administer the piggyback solution that remains in the piggyback tubing. Pinch the primary tubing closed just above the piggyback port. This'll allow the piggyback solution to drain. Watch it carefully.

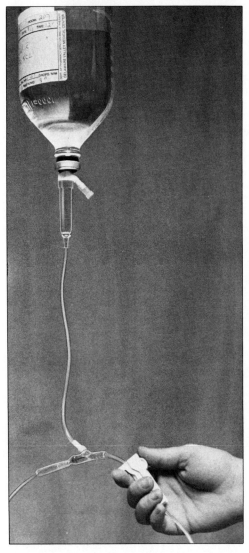

8 Open the piggyback line flow clamp. Because the minibottle's placed higher, the backcheck valve will automatically cut off the flow of *primary* solution and allow the medication to flow. (To find out how this works, see page 14.) Adjust the flow to the medication's recommended rate.

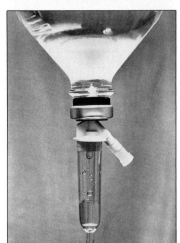

10 At the moment the tubing empties, release the pressure you've applied. This will start the primary solution running again, perhaps even filling part of the piggyback line. However, the backcheck valve will prevent the primary solution from entering the piggyback bottle.

Important: When this is done, readjust the flow rate of the primary solution to the prescribed rate; otherwise, it'll still be flowing at the piggyback rate.

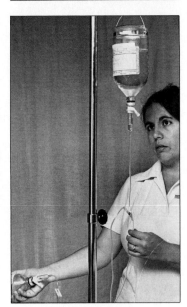

11 When you're ready to hang a *new* piggyback bottle, follow these steps to clear the tubing of air: First, disconnect the old bottle, and spike the new one. Then, open the clamp on the piggyback line, and lower the bottle below the backcheck valve. This'll cause primary fluid to run up the piggyback tubing and will expel any trapped air into the bottle. Finally, hang the piggyback container above the primary container, and adjust the flow rate.

Volume-control sets

Troubleshooting intermittent solution delivery

What problems can occur when you're administering a drug intermittently with the primary I.V. solution? And how can you prevent them? Consider these tips.

As you probably know, most drugs given intermittently run at 15- to 30-minute rates, unless otherwise specified. Double-check the drip rate, and make sure it's running as calculated.

Look at the solution. It should be clear. If precipitation's forming in the bottle or tubing, you may have reconstituted the medication incorrectly. In this case, discontinue the delivery and start again.

Make sure none of the junction sites is leaking. Check the injection port. Have you accidentally punctured the primary tubing with the secondary needle? Even if everything appears in working order, periodically double-check the entire set. If the patient moves, for example, he may dislodge a connection which will disrupt his treatment.

Understanding volume-control sets and filters

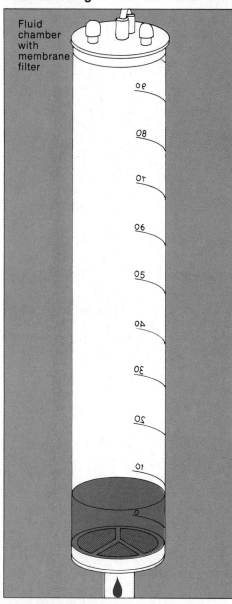

Fluid chamber with membrane filter

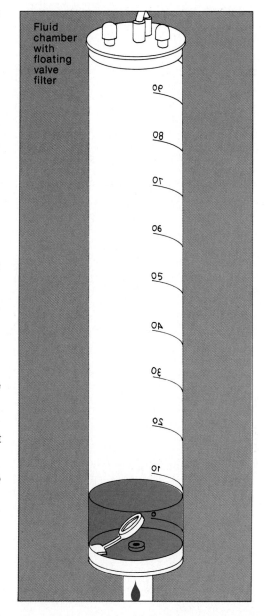

Fluid chamber with floating valve filter

Let's imagine you're faced with one of these situations: you must deliver intermittent doses of medications to a patient on I.V. therapy, or you must give medication to a child over an extended period of time. In either case, you can use a volume-control set (more commonly called a Buretrol or Soluset).

A volume-control set is an I.V. line featuring a fluid chamber. This chamber allows you to accurately deliver medication diluted in precise amounts of fluid. It's particularly useful for administering medications to a child, when even the smallest inaccuracy can be lethal.

If your patient is a child needing I.V. therapy, you'll probably use a volume-control set as a *primary* I.V. line. You'll seldom use the set for a primary I.V. line in an adult; instead you'll connect it to a secondary port of an existing line. Use the volume-control set only when it's absolutely necessary, because it's costly and easily contaminated.

Before you establish an I.V. line with a volume-control set, make sure you know which filter the set features, because it'll affect the priming procedure. You'll find either of these two filters on a volume-control set: a membrane filter or a floating valve filter. Although both filters work effectively to filter the solution, they differ in structure.

Here's how: The membrane filter, shown on the left, is rigid and remains stationary at the bottom of the fluid chamber. The floating valve filter, shown on the right, is hinged on one side. This hinge allows it to move up and down with changes in fluid chamber pressure. How do these differences affect the use of a volume-control set? Read the next few pages to find out.

Using a volume-control set with a floating valve filter

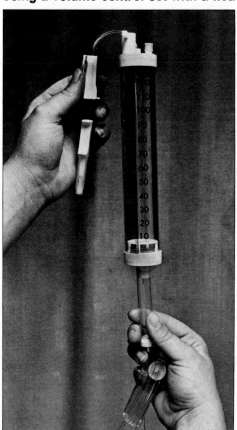

1 *Suppose your patient on I.V. therapy needs intermittent administration of an antibiotic. To give it, you could use a partial-fill piggyback set. But what if a partial-fill container's unavailable or the amount of fluid it contains (50 or 100 ml) won't suit your needs? In this case, you'd use a volume-control set.*

Open the fluid chamber air vent. Then, close the upper slide clamp, as shown here.

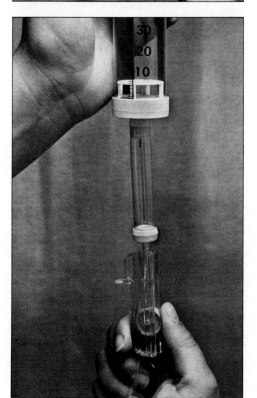

2 Now, push the lower clamp to a point just below the drip chamber and close it. Remember, don't ever leave both main clamps open. Otherwise you'll get an unregulated fluid flow.

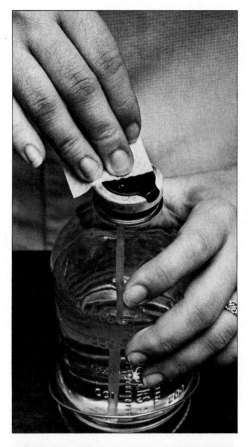

3 Use alcohol to swab the top of the container that holds the saline solution or 5% dextrose in water.

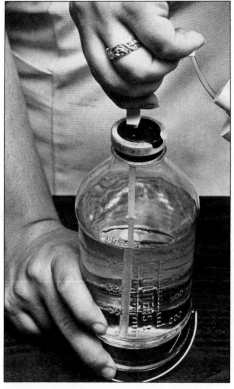

4 Remove the guard from the spike on the volume-control set, and insert the spike into the top of the container. Then, hang the set.

Volume-control sets

Using a volume-control set with a floating valve filter continued

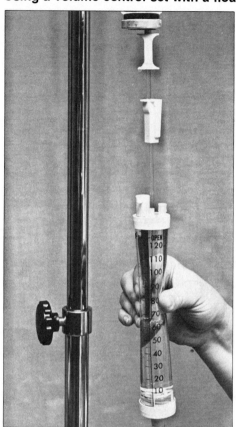

5 Open the set's upper clamp, and squeeze the fluid chamber until it's filled with approximately 30 ml of solution. Close the upper clamp.

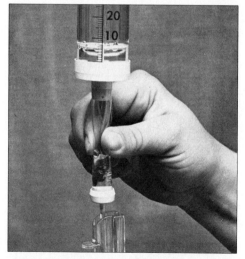

6 Now, squeeze the drip chamber until it's half full.
📧 *Nursing tip:* If the drip chamber overfills, immediately close the upper clamp and the air vent. Then, invert the fluid chamber, and squeeze the excess solution from the drip chamber back into the fluid chamber. Don't wet the air vent filter, or it may not work properly.

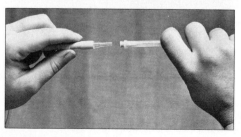

7 Continue the procedure as shown here. Remove the cover of the needle adapter, and attach a 20G 1" needle.

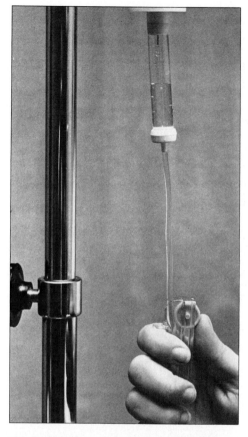

8 Open the line's lower clamp, and prime the tubing and needle. Then, close the clamp again.

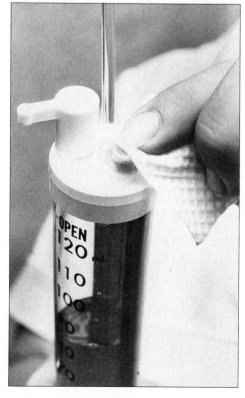

9 Now you're ready to add medication to the line. Swab the medication port on the fluid chamber with alcohol.

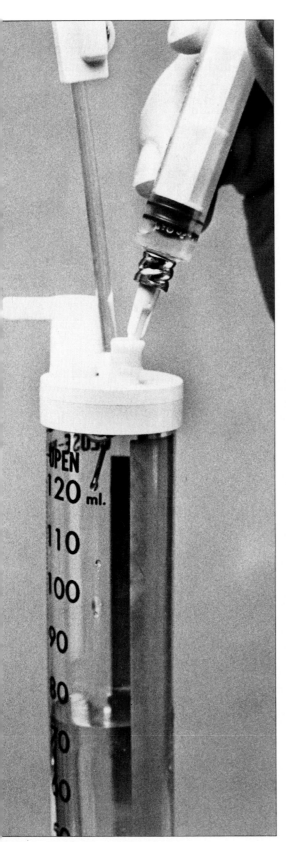

10 Draw the medication into a syringe. If the medication needs to be reconstituted, follow the procedure outlined on page 67. Then, inject it into the fluid chamber, making sure there's at least 10 ml of solution in the chamber when you do. That will make mixing easier.

Now, label the fluid chamber with the dose of medication, but don't write directly on the plastic with a felt-tip marker. If the ink's absorbed through the plastic chamber, it could contaminate the medication. Instead, write on a narrow label or tape strip.

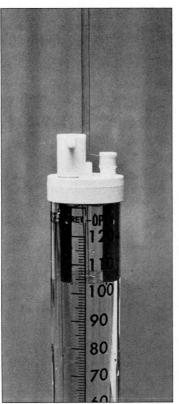

11 Open the line's upper clamp, and fill the fluid chamber with the prescribed amount of solution. Then, close the upper clamp again, and gently rotate the fluid chamber until the solution's well mixed.

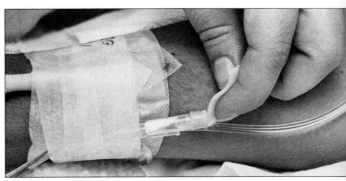

12 Swab the injection port on the primary tubing with alcohol. This step's important because the port's exposed to all types of contaminants.

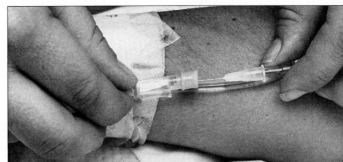

13 Insert the volume-control set needle. Use a 1" needle so you don't puncture the primary line. Secure the connection with tape.

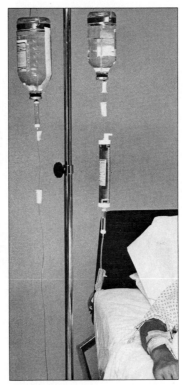

14 Turn off the primary I.V. line, or set it on a keep-vein-open (KVO) rate. Then, open the lower clamp on the volume-control set, adjust the rate, and let the medication flow. *Remember:* Document the procedure and your observations.

Volume-control sets

Using a volume-control set with a membrane filter

1 *What if the volume-control set you're using has a membrane filter instead of a floating valve filter? The procedure's the same, except for filling the drip chamber. To fill the chamber, follow these steps:*

Spike and hang the saline solution or 5% dextrose in water. Then, open the upper clamp, and let the solution drip into the fluid chamber. Don't squeeze the chamber or you'll damage the rigid membrane filter.

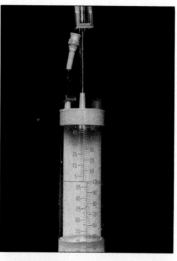

2 When approximately 30 ml of fluid have dripped down, close the upper clamp.

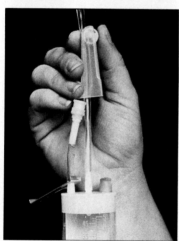

3 Then, open the lower clamp, and flatten the drip chamber. Never flatten it when the clamp's closed, because you'll rupture the membrane.

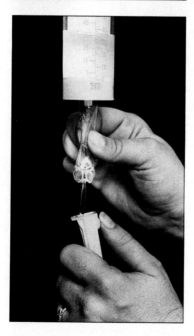

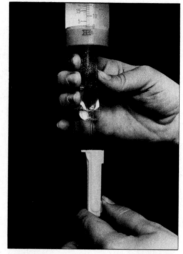

4 Keeping the chamber flattened, close the lower clamp. This will cause the chamber to retain its flattened shape. The vacuum you've created in the drip chamber will suck the solution down from the fluid chamber, and the drip chamber will return to its original shape.

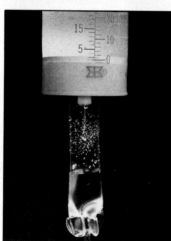

5 Repeat the procedure, nicknamed OSCAR, until the drip chamber's half full.
O—Open the lower roller clamp.
S—Squeeze the drip chamber, and maintain it while you
C—Close the lower roller clamp
A—And
R—Release your squeeze on the drip chamber.

Now that the drip chamber's partially filled, turn back to page 78. The rest of the procedure is the same as for a volume-control set with a floating valve filter.

TROUBLESHOOTING

Coping with medication problems

Many drugs cause a burning sensation when you administer them to your patient. Here are some ways you can reduce that sensation, if the doctor permits:
• Slow down the rate of infusion.
• Dilute the drug with more I.V. solution.
• Flush well after each dose to make sure no drug remains near the site.
• Add Neut to each dose, to bring the pH closer to neutral.

Remember, some drugs—nitroprusside sodium (Nipride), for example—must not be exposed to the light. In this case, cover the container with aluminum foil or a brown paper bag. Wrap the tubing in foil. Remember to put the label on the *outside* of the wrapping and to include expiration time.

I.V. bolus

Suppose one of your patients has cancer and the doctor orders the chemotherapeutic drug 5-fluorouracil (5-FU) administered by I.V. bolus. Will you know why he chose the bolus method? Suppose the patient also suffers from pulmonary congestion. Do you know what special steps to take? Suppose while you're injecting the medication, the patient goes into shock. Why has it happened, and what should you do? The following pages will answer these questions, as well as many others you may have. To find out more about giving medications by I.V. bolus, read on.

INDICATIONS/CONTRAINDICATIONS

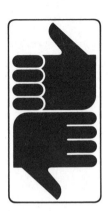

When to administer medications by I.V. bolus

As you probably know, I.V. bolus, commonly known as I.V. push, is a rapid method of administering medications intravenously.

Use I.V. bolus when:
* You need to administer medications quickly in an emergency.
* You're delivering a medication that can't be diluted; for example, Dilantin, Digoxin, Valium, Lasix, Hyperstat, many cancer chemotherapeutic drugs, and diagnostic dyes.
* You want to achieve a maximum, or peak, drug level in the patient's bloodstream.

Don't use I.V. bolus when:
* The medication you're administering—for example—an antibiotic or vitamin—must be diluted in a large-volume parenteral (LVP) before entering the bloodstream.
* The rapid administration of a medication, like KCl, could be life-threatening.

Remember, if the patient suffers from decreased cardiac output, diminished urinary output, pulmonary congestion, or systemic edema, he will have a decreased tolerance to medication. So, dilute the medication more than usual, and administer it at a slower rate.

Assembling your equipment

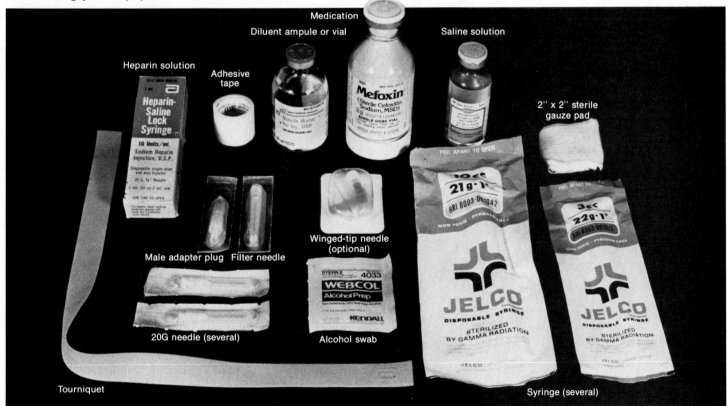

Before you begin the I.V. bolus procedure, make sure you've assembled all the necessary equipment. Much of the equipment pictured above, such as the prepping material, syringes, and needles, are common to all I.V. bolus procedures. Other equipment is used for specific I.V. bolus procedures. For example, if you do I.V. bolus by intermittent infusion, you'll need an intermittent infusion set and a heparin-filled syringe, in addition to the standard equipment.

I.V. bolus

—PATIENT PREPARATION—

Explaining I.V. bolus

Prepare the patient for I.V. bolus as follows: First, make sure he isn't allergic to the medication you plan to give. Then, describe what you're going to do. If time permits, explain why he's having drugs given to him by the I.V. bolus method. Also, alert him to the possible reactions he may experience, but don't alarm him. Answer all his questions honestly. Then, position him so he's comfortable.

Giving drugs: Some checkpoints

Planning to give your patient medication? Before you take it to his bedside, ask yourself these questions:
• What's this drug's action?
• Through which routes can this drug be given?
• What side effects can the patient have from this drug?
• Which other drugs aid, or potentiate, this drug's effectiveness?
• Which other drugs hinder, or antagonize, this drug's effectiveness?
• Will other factors in the patient's condition affect the drug's action?
• Which diluent should be used with this drug?
• How much diluent should be used with this drug?
• What's the required amount of time to safely inject the prescribed dosage of this drug?
  Important: Anytime you have questions about the drug or its prescribed dosage, consult a reference book, like the NURSE'S GUIDE TO DRUGS.

Timing the injection

Use a wristwatch with a second hand to time all I.V. bolus injections. Avoid the temptation to rush administration. Injections usually take from 1 to 30 minutes. To figure how much of the medication should be given per minute, simply take the total amount and divide it by the prescribed time required. Before actually doing an I.V. bolus, practice administering the medication at the prescribed rate. This'll increase your confidence and make working with the patient easier.

Administering drugs by I.V. bolus

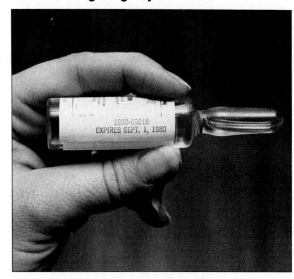

1 *Before delivering a drug by the I.V. bolus method, make sure you have the medication order correct.* Double-check the drug label to confirm that it matches the doctor's medication order. Also check the expiration date to make sure the drug's not outdated.

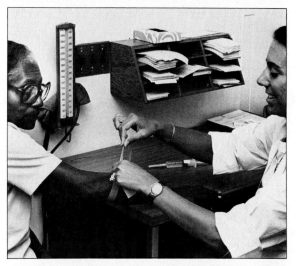

2 Now, apply a tourniquet, and select the largest suitable vein. Choose a site with the patient's comfort and your convenience in mind. Remember, a large vein will provide greater dilution, thereby minimizing any irritation from the drug.

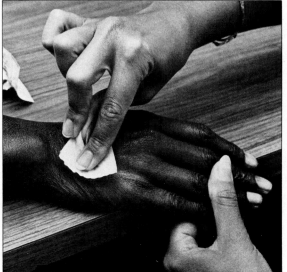

3 Now, prep the site as you would for venipuncture, using a swab to apply alcohol in a circular motion. Refer back to page 30 to refresh your memory on the entire prepping procedure.

As an optional next step, many nurses, including the one shown here, insert a small winged-tip needle into the bolus site so they can inject the medication through it. What are the advantages to this? First, the small size of the winged-tip needle lessens the risk of collapsing the vein and causing trauma; second, the winged-tip needle is much more stable than a syringe needle and is less likely to damage the vein.

4 Do you need to reconstitute the medication before you administer it? If so, follow the procedure outlined on page 67. Then, draw up the medication through a filter needle, remembering to replace the filter needle with a regular needle afterward. Invert the syringe, and tap out any trapped air bubbles.

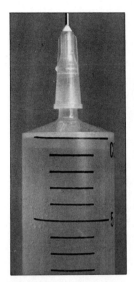

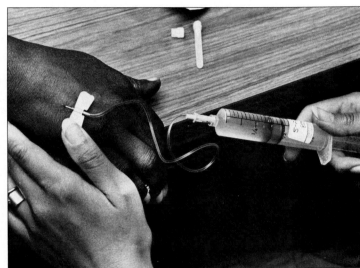

7 Before you begin injecting the drug, steady your hand on the patient's arm or some nearby support.

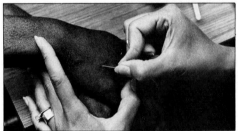

5 If your patient's vein is prominent, enter it in one step (direct method), inserting the needle at a 30° angle. When you do, make sure the needle bevel is at least ¼" inside the vein. Don't use the direct method if the vein's small. If you do, you'll risk passing the needle right through it. Instead, use the two-step, or indirect, method of venipunture described on page 32.

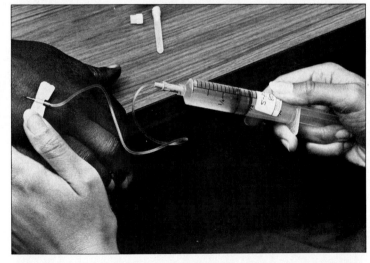

8 Now, remove the tourniquet, and begin injecting the drug bolus at the prescribed rate. For more details on how to time injections, see page 82.

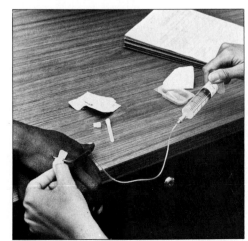

6 Now, pull back on the syringe, and check for blood backflow. This will insure that the needle's securely in the vein.

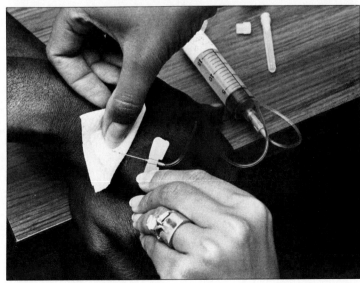

9 When you've finished, wait for a slight blood backflow before removing the needle. This way you're sure the needle's still in the vein and there's no threat of drug extravasation. Withdraw the needle. Immediately apply pressure to the site with a 2" x 2" sterile gauze pad for 1 minute. Use a narrow strip of adhesive (if necessary) to hold the gauze in place.

I.V. bolus

Administering an I.V. bolus through a primary line

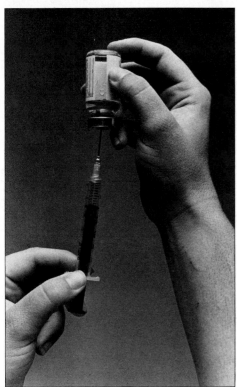

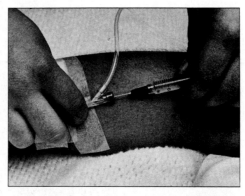

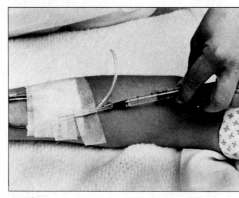

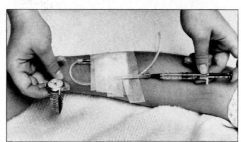

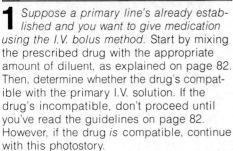

1 *Suppose a primary line's already established and you want to give medication using the I.V. bolus method.* Start by mixing the prescribed drug with the appropriate amount of diluent, as explained on page 82. Then, determine whether the drug's compatible with the primary I.V. solution. If the drug's incompatible, don't proceed until you've read the guidelines on page 82. However, if the drug *is* compatible, continue with this photostory.

2 First, swab the injection port with alcohol. Then, insert the needle into the injection port. If the port has an *O* marked on it, inject the medication *within this circle* or the port will leak.

📨 *Nursing tip:* Whenever you're inserting or withdrawing a needle from an injection port, hold the port steady with your free hand. This way you won't accidentally dislodge the cannula.

Before continuing, close the roller clamp.

3 Draw back on the syringe to check for blood backflow. Make sure the I.V. needle's properly placed in the vein. Make sure there's no sign of infiltration.

4 Inject the medication at the prescribed rate. When you're finished, open the roller clamp. If the medication's one that tends to irritate the vein, let the I.V. fluid run rapidly through the line for about a minute. This'll help dilute the medication. Then, open the flow clamp, and adjust the flow rate.

Using an intermittent-infusion set

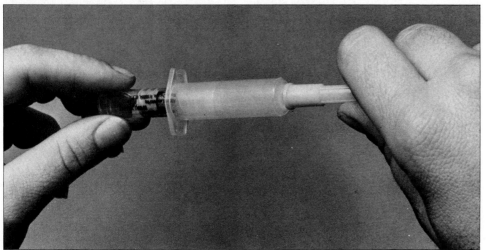

1 *Instead of connecting your patient to a primary I.V. line, you can use an intermittent-infusion set to administer drugs, collect blood samples, give intermittent transfusions, or get circulatory access in emergencies. Besides being convenient, the set prevents fluid overloading and allows the patient to move around freely.*

Begin the procedure by preparing a heparin flush. Recent studies show that as little as 10 units of heparin per ml of saline solution is adequate. Most hospitals advocate using 100 units per ml of saline solution. Either way, draw the heparin into a syringe from a single- or multidose vial, or use a prefilled heparin syringe.

As you may know, the multidose vial is the least expensive, but it increases the risk of contamination.

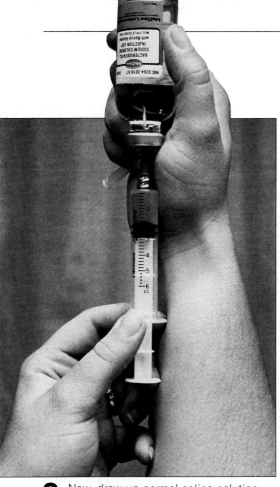

2 Now, draw up normal saline solution into a syringe, as the nurse is doing in the above photo.

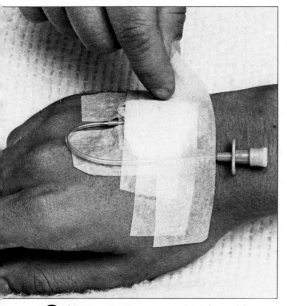

3 Next, prepare your patient for venipuncture, as explained on pages 29 and 30. Insert an intermittent-infusion set as you would a winged-tip needle, and tape it securely. However, secure the set's injection port as far from the venipuncture site as possible. This will reduce your chances of moving the needle during the injection.

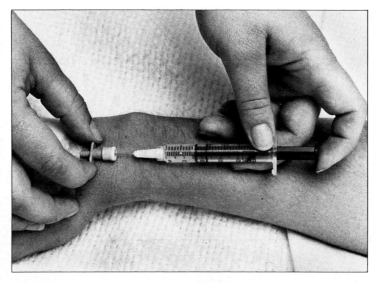

4 Swab the injection port with alcohol or, even better, iodophor prep.
    Now, insert the needle of the medication syringe into the port. Make sure you use a 1" needle. Anything longer might pierce the catheter. First, check for blood backflow. Then, inject the medication at the recommended rate.

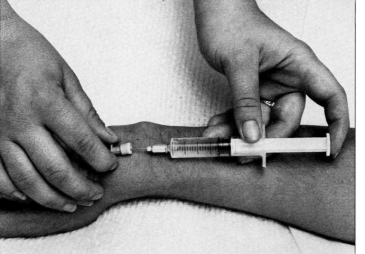

5 Now, depending on your hospital's policy, follow the drug injection with one or both of these steps:
    First, withdraw the medication syringe, and insert the needle of the saline-filled syringe in its place. Flush out any medication that remains.

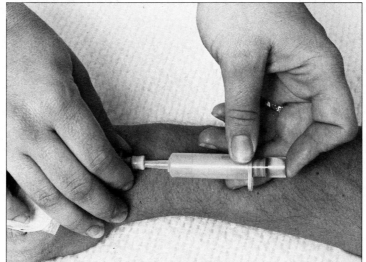

6 Then, swab the port with alcohol or iodophor prep. Insert the heparin-filled syringe, and inject the heparinized solution. This'll keep the tubing patent.
    Now you're ready to use the intermittent-infusion set again when you need to.

I.V. bolus

Coping with incompatibilities

1 *If the drug you're administering is incompatible with the primary solution, follow these steps:*
  Mix the drug with a diluent, and draw it up into a syringe. Then, draw saline solution into two other syringes.

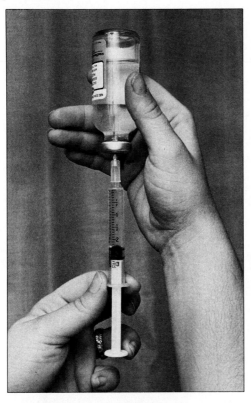

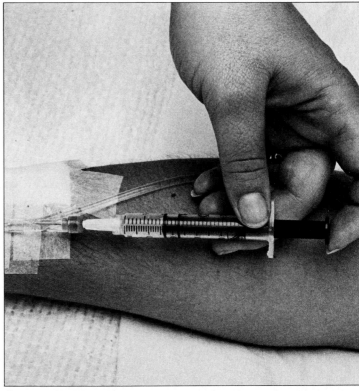

3 Then, follow the same procedure for a compatible drug injection, from swabbing the port with alcohol through injecting the medication. Don't open the roller clamp until you've flushed the tubing with the remaining saline-filled syringe.

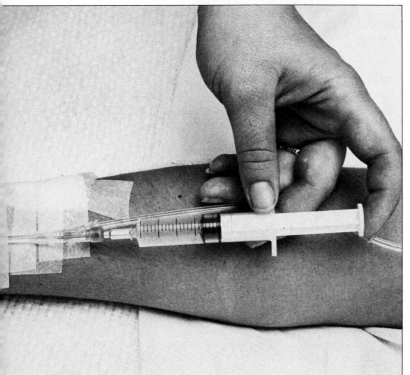

2 Next, close the roller clamp. Insert the needle of one of the saline-filled syringes into the line's secondary port. After checking for blood backflow, flush the tubing with saline solution.

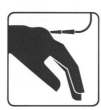

___COMPLICATIONS___

Watching for adverse reactions

Remember, when you give a drug by the I.V. bolus method, it'll have an immediate effect. Pay special attention to the patient's reaction. If he's able to respond, ask him how he feels. Listen to his complaints. He may be experiencing side effects; for example, chills; nausea; or localized pain, burning, or itching. If he is, stop the drug immediately, check his vital signs, and call the doctor.
  Be alert for possible *speed shock*—the body's reaction to an injection of a foreign substance into the circulation. When a drug's injected too rapidly, it can cause the blood's plasma concentration to reach toxic proportions. These toxins will then infiltrate the blood-rich organs, for example, the brain and the heart. This may cause syncope, shock, or cardiac arrest.

Using the male adapter plug

1 *If you want to discontinue I.V. therapy but keep the catheter patent for occasional injections, use a male adapter plug. Here's how:*

First, check for blood backflow by lowering the I.V. container or using a saline-filled syringe. Then, prepare another syringe, filled with heparin solution. Prime the male adapter plug with heparin.

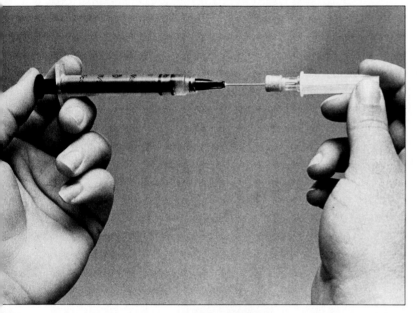

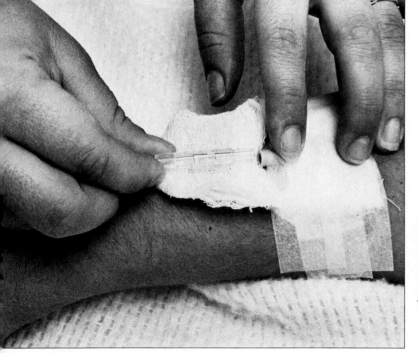

2 Place a 2" x 2" sterile gauze pad or an alcohol swab just under the catheter hub. Then, close the roller clamp on the I.V. line, and disconnect the line from the catheter hub.

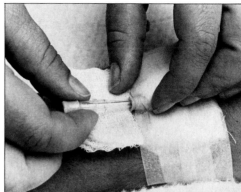

3 Remove the adapter plug's cap, and insert the plug into the catheter hub.

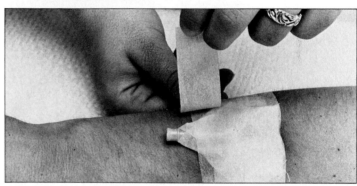

4 Secure the male adapter plug with tape. Don't forget to incorporate daily redressing of the male adapter plug into your care plan.

Using the obturator

Let's imagine you're caring for a patient on I.V. therapy, and you have orders to disconnect the I.V. temporarily so he can be transported to another department. Keep the catheter patent by using a sterile disposable obturator. Simply insert the obturator tip into the injection port, and turn it until it locks in place. Secure the obturator with tape. Now the catheter's protected from contamination.

Remember: Never use the same obturator twice. It must be sterile when it's inserted in the port.

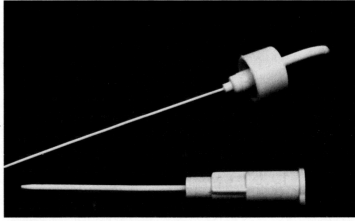

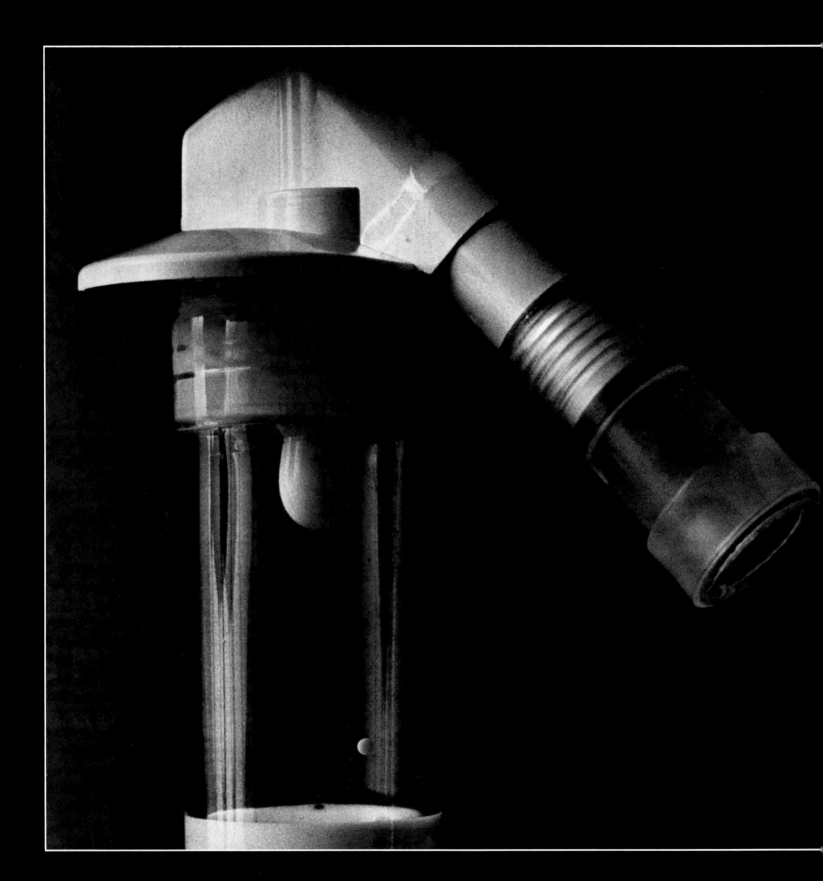

Giving Parenteral Nutrition

Hyperalimentation

I.V. fat emulsions

Hyperalimentation

Suppose you're caring for a patient with severe chest and arm burns. And the doctor orders hyperalimentation therapy. Do you know what's expected of you? For example, what role you play in the various insertion procedures? How to manage various insertion sites? How to change tubing and dressing? If you're uncertain, read the next few pages. From them, you'll find out the answers to these and other questions about hyperalimentation.

---INDICATIONS/CONTRAINDICATIONS---

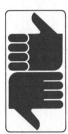

When to administer hyperalimentation

You'll administer hyperalimentation by deep vein to the patient who needs nutrients for growth and development. The doctor will order it when the patient can't get adequate nutrition with a standard diet or through oral or enteral feeding.

Don't give it to patients who:
• Are terminally ill and have had all therapy discontinued
• Suffer from bleeding abnormalities or hypercoagulation
• Have an obstructed or partially thrombosed superior vena cava.

Special consideration:
If the doctor orders, the patient who's threatened by renal or hepatic failure can receive a specially prepared hyperalimentation solution.

Assembling hyperalimentation equipment

One of your important responsibilities in hyperalimentation therapy is assembling the equipment prior to insertion. Make sure everything's in working order. *Remember:* Sterile conditions are particularly crucial in hyperalimentation therapy. Observe strict aseptic technique whenever you're handling the equipment.

Hyperalimentation solution

Hyperalimentation tubing (with 0.22 micron filter)

Sterile gloves

Alcohol swabs

Sterile hemostat

Antimicrobial ointment

Iodine solution

4" x 4" sterile gauze pads

Inside-the-needle catheter (INC)

Tincture of benzoin

Luer-Tip syringe

Sterile scissors

Anesthetic

Suture material

Hemostat

Acetone solution

Saline solution

Air-occlusive tape

Adhesive tape

5% dextrose in water

Sterile gown and mask (optional)

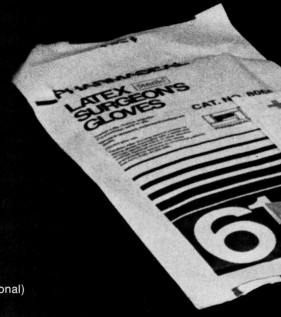

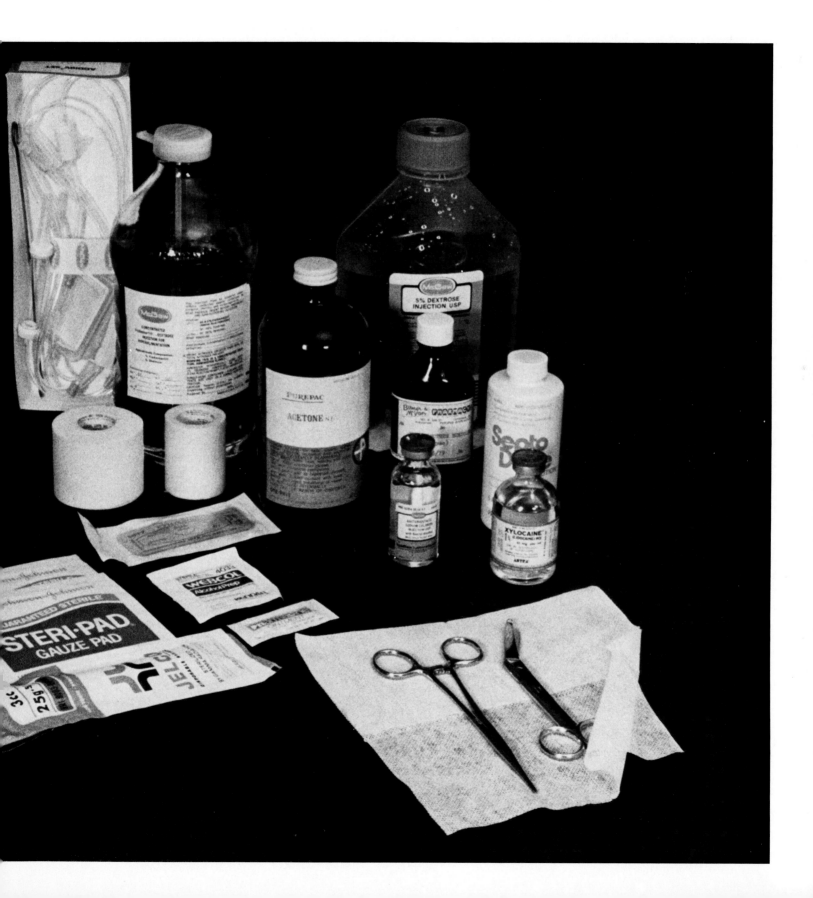

Hyperalimentation

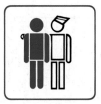

Explaining hyperalimentation

The idea of hyperalimentation may be so new to your patient that he'll probably be frightened about the prospect. To help him, explain in words he can understand:

- the purpose or goal of the procedure
- the positions he'll be in
- the insertion technique
- the pumps and their alarm systems, if you're using them

- the tubing, filter, and dressing change procedures.
  Encourage your patient to ask questions, and answer them honestly. Remember, to the patient, I.V. therapy may look more dangerous than it actually is. If he understands the procedure, and you assure him that you'll take special care of him, you can alleviate much of his stress.
  Don't forget, the patient will probably have to sign a consent form before a central line can be inserted.

Selecting the insertion site

To administer hyperalimentation therapy, the doctor may use either a direct central line, a central line through a peripheral vein, or a central line through the jugular vein. Each site has its own benefits and drawbacks, as the following chart shows, and the selection is largely a matter of the doctor's preference.

We'll discuss these insertion sites for hyperalimentation therapy, but they can also be used, at separate times, for:
- CVP monitoring (see page 140)
- long-term intravenous therapy
- repeated withdrawal of representative mixed venous blood specimens
- rapid infusion of large amounts of fluid.

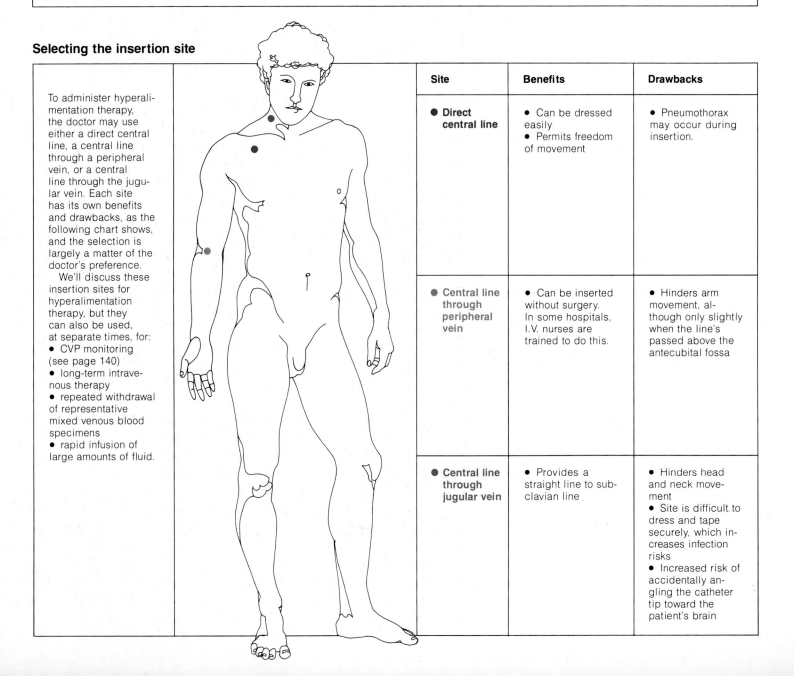

Site	Benefits	Drawbacks
● Direct central line	● Can be dressed easily ● Permits freedom of movement	● Pneumothorax may occur during insertion.
● Central line through peripheral vein	● Can be inserted without surgery. In some hospitals, I.V. nurses are trained to do this.	● Hinders arm movement, although only slightly when the line's passed above the antecubital fossa
● Central line through jugular vein	● Provides a straight line to subclavian line	● Hinders head and neck movement ● Site is difficult to dress and tape securely, which increases infection risks ● Increased risk of accidentally angling the catheter tip toward the patient's brain

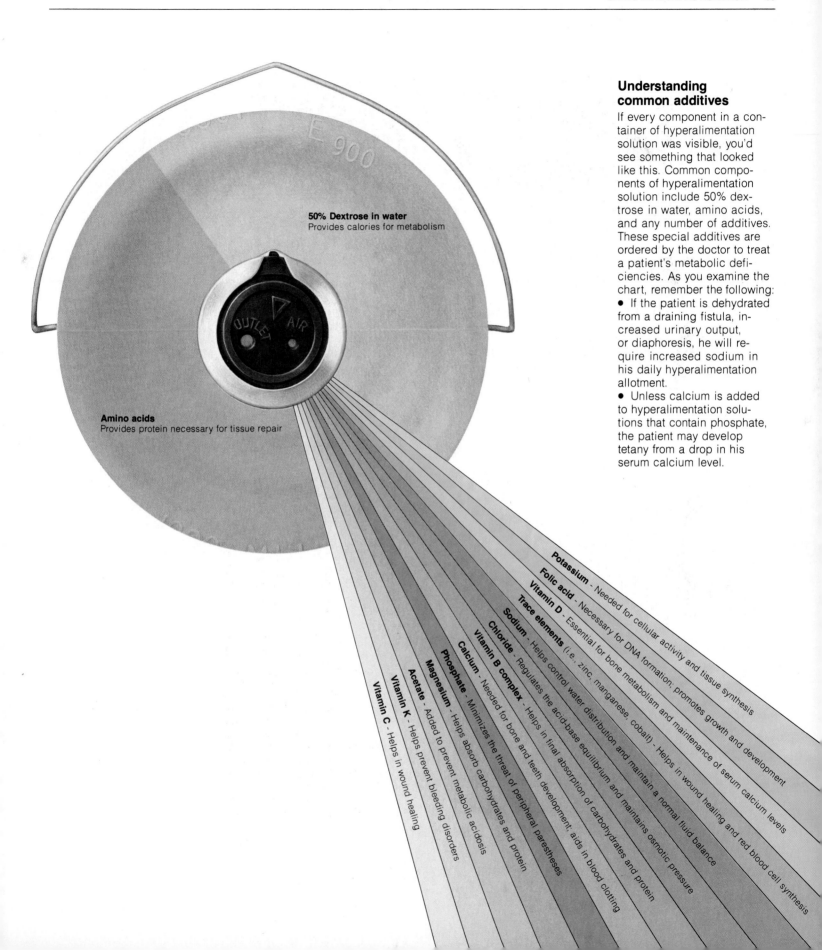

50% Dextrose in water
Provides calories for metabolism

Amino acids
Provides protein necessary for tissue repair

Understanding common additives

If every component in a container of hyperalimentation solution was visible, you'd see something that looked like this. Common components of hyperalimentation solution include 50% dextrose in water, amino acids, and any number of additives. These special additives are ordered by the doctor to treat a patient's metabolic deficiencies. As you examine the chart, remember the following:
• If the patient is dehydrated from a draining fistula, increased urinary output, or diaphoresis, he will require increased sodium in his daily hyperalimentation allotment.
• Unless calcium is added to hyperalimentation solutions that contain phosphate, the patient may develop tetany from a drop in his serum calcium level.

Potassium - Needed for cellular activity and tissue synthesis
Folic acid - Necessary for DNA formation; promotes growth and development
Vitamin D - Essential for bone metabolism and maintenance of serum calcium levels
Trace elements (i.e., zinc, manganese, cobalt) - Helps in wound healing and red blood cell synthesis
Sodium - Helps control water distribution and maintain a normal fluid balance
Chloride - Regulates the acid-base equilibrium and maintains osmotic pressure
Vitamin B complex - Helps in final absorption of carbohydrates and protein; aids in blood clotting
Calcium - Needed for bone and teeth development; aids in blood clotting
Phosphate - Minimizes the threat of peripheral parestheses
Magnesium - Helps absorb carbohydrates and protein
Acetate - Added to prevent metabolic acidosis
Vitamin K - Helps prevent bleeding disorders
Vitamin C - Helps in wound healing

Hyperalimentation

Helping the doctor insert a direct central line

1 *Suppose you're going to assist the doctor as he inserts a direct central line into the patient's subclavian vein. Do you know what's expected of you? Begin by checking the patient's wristband to verify identification. Then, match her name with the name on the hyperalimentation container. If identification's correct, start the procedure.*

First, if your patient's male, check to see if his chest hair covers the intended venipuncture site. If it does, shave it off in an area about 5″ around the site.

Then, place the patient in the Trendelenburg position, as shown here. This position encourages the vein to dilate and fill, reducing the risk of air embolism.

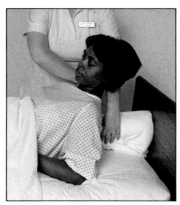

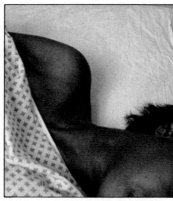

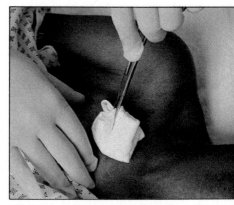

2 Now, place a rolled towel or blanket lengthwise between her shoulders, as shown here, to further encourage vein distention.

3 To minimize site contamination and make the vein more accessible, turn the patient's head away from the site. Your hospital may advocate slipping a mask over the patient's nose and mouth. Explain to her why it's necessary. But don't apply the mask if the patient has trouble breathing, like this one.

4 Wearing sterile gloves, clean the insertion site and an area about 5″ around it. To do this motion, as this illustration shows. Then, replace the used gauze pad with a dry one, and repeat the process twice to remove all dirt and perspiration.

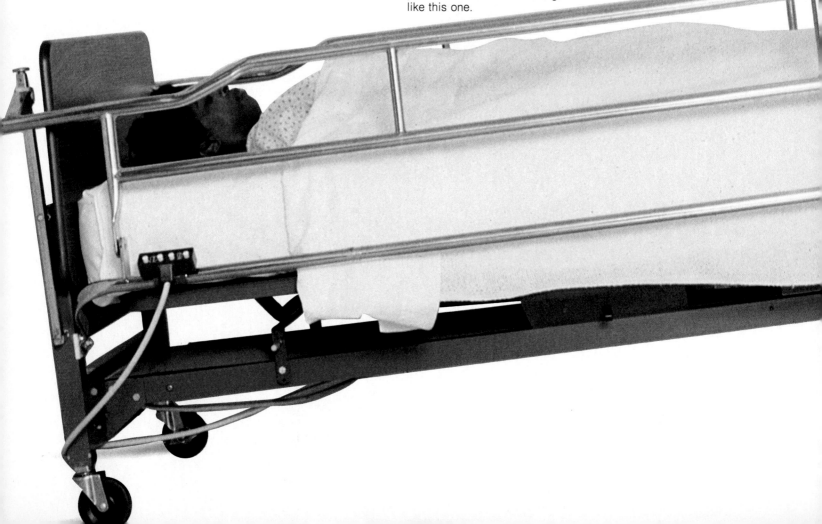

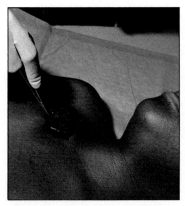

5 Now, paint the site with povidine-iodine. Let it dry naturally for at least 2 minutes.

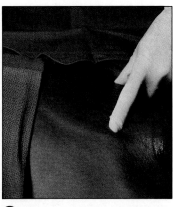

6 Surround the site with sterile drapes. Have sterile gloves ready. *Remember:* The doctor will maintain sterile technique throughout the procedure.

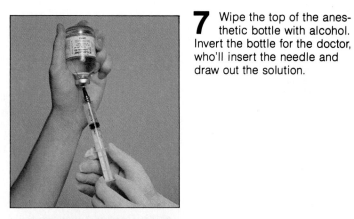

7 Wipe the top of the anesthetic bottle with alcohol. Invert the bottle for the doctor, who'll insert the needle and draw out the solution.

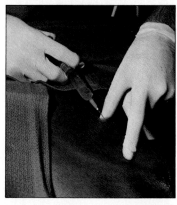

8 The doctor will then inject the local anesthetic into the site, as this photo shows.

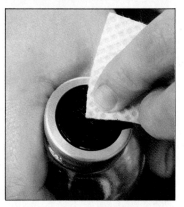

9 While he's doing this, remove the protective cap from the container of 5% dextrose in water. If the solution's in a bottle, wipe the top with an alcohol swab.

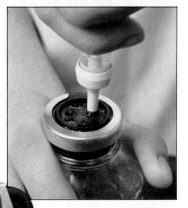

10 Now, close the tubing's roller clamp to prevent a rush of air into the tube when you insert the spike. Remove the spike guard. Push the spike into the bottle stopper or the bag port. Then, invert the container and suspend it.

Hyperalimentation

Helping the doctor insert a direct central line continued

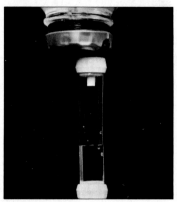

11 Squeeze the drip chamber until it's half full. If you accidentally overfill it, you won't be able to see the drip action. Remedy such a mistake by inverting the container and squeezing some of the solution back into it.

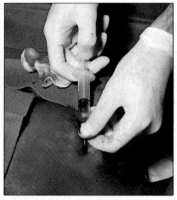

12 This photo shows the doctor inserting the needle. While he's doing this, continue with your work.

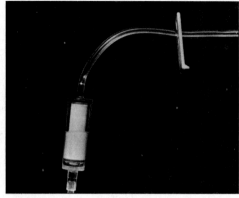

13 To reduce the risk of an air embolism, add an air-eliminating filter (0.22 micron) to the far end of the tubing. Open the slide clamp. Run the solution into the filter until it's completely filled.

Get ready for the doctor to insert the catheter. As he does, monitor the patient's heart rhythm closely. If the patient shows signs of new arrhythmias, the catheter tip may be irritating her heart and may need adjustment.

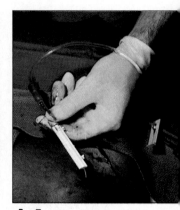

14 After the insertion, the doctor will hold the end of the catheter hub and connect the tubing. Then, the doctor may suture the catheter to keep it in place, as this photo shows.

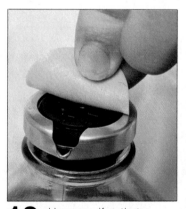

18 However, if catheter placement's correct, you can hang the hyperalimentation solution and connect it to the line without endangering the patient.

Here's how: Remove the protective cap from the container. Swab the bottle stopper or the bag port with alcohol.

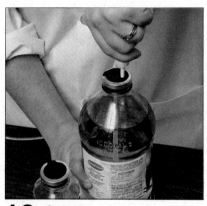

19 Close the roller clamp. Unhook the container of 5% dextrose in water. Withdraw the spike, and insert it into the container of hyperalimentation solution.

Important: Make sure the solution's been standing at room temperature for 1 hour.

Hang the container. Then, adjust the flow rate. Now you're ready for final taping.

Important: Before you document the procedure, double-check the solution, flow rate, tubing connections, and the insertion site. Then, document your observations, following the charting tips on page 43. Double-check the set-up periodically.

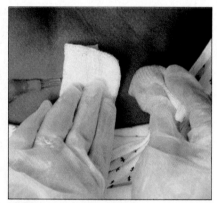

20 Proper dressing and taping of a hyperalimentation insertion site is crucial to the therapy's success. To do this correctly, begin by putting on a pair of sterile gloves. Then, place a 2" x 2" sterile gauze pad on the insertion site. Apply a generous border of benzoin around the dressing to help it adhere and to prevent tissue breakdown. Let it dry for at least 1 minute. (Remember, it'll remain tacky to the touch.) Don't hasten the drying process by fanning the site with your hands. When that's completed, take off your gloves and discard them.

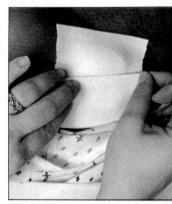

21 Keep the patient's head turned away so she doesn't breathe on the insertion site. Apply enough protective elastic bandage to insure an air-occlusive dressing. Make sure the bandage covers the entire catheter but not the connection hub. This'll allow you to change the tubing easily.

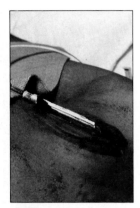

15 Begin dressing the site by applying antimicrobial ointment, as shown here. Cover the insertion site with a 2" x 2" sterile gauze pad. Make sure the needle guard's securely fastened down.

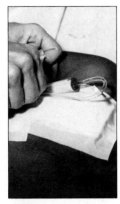

16 Use adhesive tape to secure the edges of the dressing. Remember, this dressing is a temporary one, to cover the site for an X-ray.

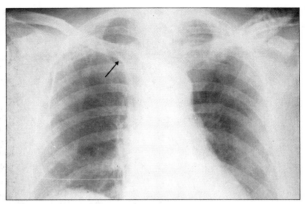

17 Place the patient in the high Fowler's position so she can be X-rayed for proper catheter placement. If improperly placed, a catheter can damage one of the patient's lungs and cause a pneumothorax. Watch for signs of pneumothorax; for example, labored breathing and chest pains. Have a chest tube handy in case the doctor needs to insert one.

Suppose the X-ray shows that the catheter's improperly placed. The doctor will adjust the catheter's position or withdraw it and repeat the procedure.

Maintaining the central line

Infection can seriously threaten the health of your patient receiving a hyperalimentation solution. The solution's high sugar content and the patient's weakened state make the following conditions particularly likely: *Candida* (fungal), *Staph aureus, Staph epidermidis,* or *Klebsiella.* You can minimize this risk by observing strict aseptic technique.

Here are some additional precautions:
• Never take a blood sample, do a CVP reading, or piggyback any solution on a hyperalimentation line.
• If any part of the equipment becomes contaminated, or the catheter develops a leak, change the entire I.V. setup.
• Watch for signs of infection: redness, swelling, oozing, pus, or a sudden temperature rise. If you spot them, notify the doctor immediately.
• Also watch for signs of thrombosis. Call the doctor if the patient's experiencing pain or soreness in his chest, shoulder, or neck; you observe swelling in his catheterized arm; or you observe neck vein distention.

Suppose the doctor confirms thrombosis. He'll remove the catheter and may order anticoagulant therapy.
• Always infuse the hyperalimentation solution at a constant rate, or you may cause metabolic complications: for example, hyperglycemia or hyperosmolarity. Avoid interrupting treatment to feed in other fluids. Don't infuse the solution too rapidly, or you risk causing a fluid overload. Never attempt to catch up on feedings that are behind schedule.

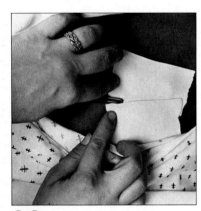

22 Now, you're ready to seal the dressing with 1" wide adhesive tape or several wide strips of air-occlusive tape. Cut a ½" slit in the tape's center. Then, position the tape so that the catheter rests in the slit, as this photo shows. Now, you won't loosen the dressing when you change the tubing.

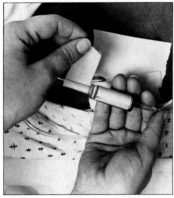

23 Secure all tubing connections with adhesive tape, to prevent accidental tube separation and to protect the patient against air embolism or blood loss. Anchor the filter to minimize catheter tension.

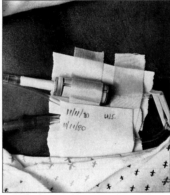

24 Now, label the dressing tag with the following: date and time of catheter insertion, the initials of the doctor who inserted it, and the date the dressing was applied. Tape the tag to the dressing. Document all relevant information.

One further precaution: If your patient has a neck wound or a tracheostomy, place a 3" x 5" sterile drape over the subclavian dressing to protect it from contamination.

◉ *Nursing tip:* Whenever you assist with a central line insertion, remove the soiled dressings from the patient's room as you leave.

Hyperalimentation

Inserting a central line peripherally

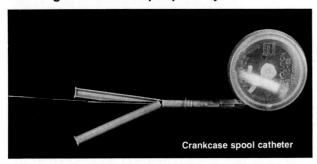

Crankcase spool catheter

What are the benefits of inserting a central line through a peripheral vein? Do you understand your role in this new procedure? If you have any questions, read this page.

Sooner or later, you'll probably administer hyperalimentation to a patient through a peripherally inserted central line. If you work in one of the few select hospitals that are doing this procedure, you're familiar with the new type of catheter being used. Because this catheter is inserted nonsurgically, you may be responsible for inserting and maintaining the line.

If you are, begin the procedure as you would any venipuncture. Wash your hands, and assemble all the equipment you'll need. In the photo above, you'll see the special silicone catheter you'll be inserting. This catheter is elastic and highly flexible. It's wound on a crankcase spool to make insertion easier. Familiarize yourself with how it works by reading the manufacturer's instructions.

Now, prep the patient's skin, and dilate the vein in the usual manner. Position his head down, and toward the insertion site, to facilitate correct catheter placement. Perform venipuncture, using the indirect method. Then, turn the crankcase spool clockwise to feed the catheter into the vein. *Note:* Each revolution of the spool feeds 5" of catheter into the vein. Estimate how many revolutions are needed to cover the distance between the insertion site and the subclavian vein.

When the catheter's inserted, disassemble the crankcase following the manufacturer's instructions. Then, get an X-ray to confirm correct catheter placement. When you're sure it's placed correctly, dress and tape the site as you would for any venipuncture.

A catheter as flexible as this one has many advantages: it allows greater arm movement, is less irritating, and minimizes the risk of thrombosis. However, it can cause the following complications:
- *Occlusion.* A common risk, which you can counter by flushing the peripheral line with dilute streptokinase, a thrombolytic enzyme.
- *Phlebitis.* Also a common risk but not always a serious one. If the patient receives proper treatment, you may be able to leave the catheter in place.
- *Infection.* Usually evidenced by purulent drainage at the insertion site, accompanied by an elevated white blood cell count. If you suspect an infection, culture the site. The doctor may want to order an antibiotic. In severe cases, he may order removal of the line.
- *Catheter sensitivity.* Evidenced by fever and sometimes phlebitis. In most cases, the doctor will let the reaction run its course. But if the patient's body continues to resist the catheter, he may order removal of the line.

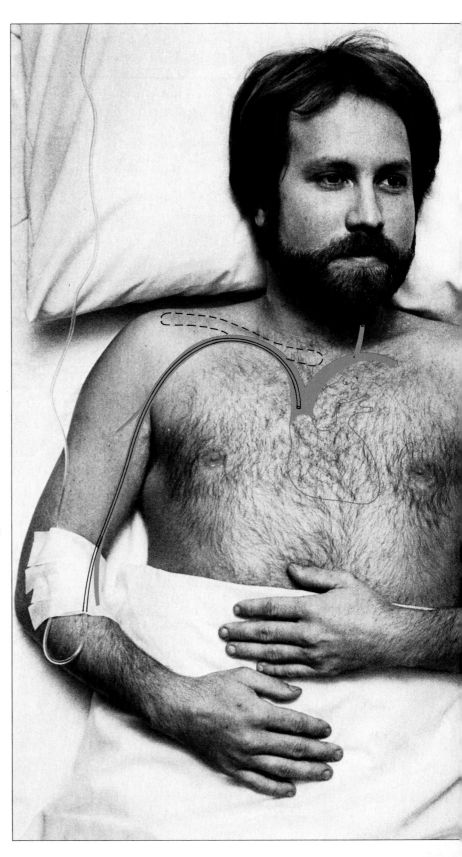

Maintaining a jugular line

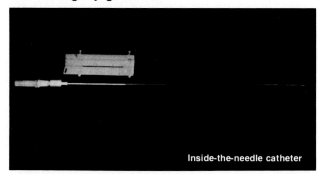

Inside-the-needle catheter

Under what circumstances will the doctor insert a central line through a patient's jugular vein? Do you know what equipment he'll need and how you'll assist him? Learn the answers by reading this page.

Some doctors use this vein for a central line because it's easily accessible. Other doctors will use it only when the chest and arm are inaccessible because of injury, burns, fat deposits, or repeated venipuncture sticks.

The jugular vein should never be used if the patient suffers from any neurologic disorder, a thoracicoaortic aneurysm, or a severe atherosclerotic vascular disease.

Let's suppose the doctor's inserting a jugular line for hyperalimentation or CVP monitoring. Chances are, he'll use the right internal jugular vein, because it leads directly to the superior vena cava. The left internal jugular vein also provides a route to the superior vena cava, but it's more hazardous since the vein's located near the patient's thoracic duct. (The thoracic duct, if damaged, could lead to chylothorax.)

The external jugular veins are rarely used for hyperalimentation or CVP monitoring, because they form sharp angles where they meet the subclavian vein, making catheter passage difficult.

When you assist the doctor with a jugular insertion, gather the equipment he'll need for a central line, plus an assortment of 8" to 12" long radiopaque catheters.

Then, position the patient flat on his back in the Trendelenburg position. This'll expose the sternal and the claviculate portion of the sternocleidomastoid muscle, which the doctor must locate to find the correct insertion site. Turn the patient's head away from the selected site. Place a pillow under the patient's shoulder, to extend his neck.

Now, prep the entire right side of the patient's neck, as you would the chest for a direct subclavian procedure. The doctor will then inject an anesthetic, raise a wheal, and advance the needle portion of the INC into the anterior cervical space. After that, he'll feed the catheter into the patient's internal jugular vein and from there into the subclavian vein or right atrium. Then, he'll withdraw the obturator and the needle, and fasten (possibly suture) the plastic needle guard in place.

When that's completed, dress the insertion site almost like you'd dress a direct subclavian site. In this case, however, loop the catheter loosely over the patient's ear and then back toward the site before taping it. Doing so will allow the patient to move his head freely.

Now, help the patient into a high Fowler's position, which will prevent hematoma formation. Get a chest X-ray to confirm correct placement of the catheter tip.

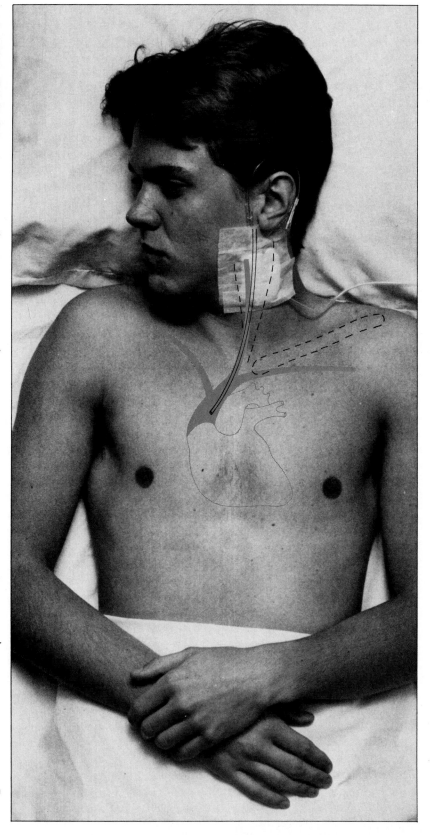

Hyperalimentation

Administering protein-sparing solutions

You don't always need a central line to meet your patient's nutritional needs. If you're administering a protein-sparing solution, you can deliver it through a peripheral vein without causing irritation. Here's why:

Protein-sparing solutions contain the same amounts of electrolytes, vitamins, and minerals as hyperalimentation solutions but about one half the amount of amino acids. They also contain varying amounts of dextrose, up to 10%. In many cases, a protein-sparing solution is supplemented with an I.V. fat emulsion, to provide calories for the patient.
• The doctor will probably order protein-sparing solutions for patients who suffer acute trauma, have major surgery, receive radiation therapy, or receive chemotherapy.

• He won't order it for patients who suffer from cardiac failure, renal or hepatic failure, or shock.

Always infuse protein-sparing solution in a peripheral vein, using the same aseptic technique used for central hyperalimentation therapy. For best results, maintain an even flow rate.

Like any potent drug admixture, protein-sparing solutions can cause the following complications: phlebitis (both chemical and septic), or subcutaneous tissue infiltration, with possible necrosis and sloughing.

To prevent such complications, observe the site for signs of tenderness, redness, or edema. If they're present, withdraw the catheter and change the site. Notify the doctor, and document your observations.

Planning day-to-day care

To provide good care for the patient receiving hyperalimentation, you should:
• Check and document his vital signs at least once every 4 hours.
• Test urine sugar, acetone, and specific gravity every 6 hours.

Dipstick test results will show whether or not the patient's tolerating the extra carbohydrate he's receiving. In many cases, the patient will show a sugar level as high as 2+ during the first few days of treatment. But if his sugar level goes beyond 2+ and remains high, notify the doctor. He may increase the insulin level in the hyperalimentation solution.

Important: Suppose your patient's sugar level is normal and then suddenly becomes elevated. He may be developing an infection. Notify the doctor promptly and document your findings.

If the test shows the patient has a high acetone concentration, he may need protein supplements. Consult the doctor.
• Weigh the patient at the same time daily, making sure he wears the same clothing. By doing so, you can better evaluate his caloric and fluid needs.
• Keep accurate intake and output records, as well as calorie counts.
• Monitor the patient's fluid and elec-

trolyte status, including tests for phosphate, magnesium, osmolarity, blood sugar, blood urea nitrogen (BUN), and creatinine levels. Because the hyperalimentation solution has so many components that affect blood differently, you must make accurate studies and keep up-to-date records.
• Provide good mouth care. If you don't, your patient may develop parotitis, glossy tongue, or oral lesions. To insure good oral hygiene, give the patient flavored mouthwash and flavored lip balm.
• Remember, while your patient's receiving hyperalimentation solution, he may imagine he tastes or smells food. The longer he remains on this therapy, the greater this phenomenon may become. If it's a problem, try managing it as follows: First, explain to the patient that such strange sensations are common. Distract him at mealtimes by encouraging him to ambulate or attend to personal grooming chores. Ask the doctor if the patient can chew or suck on hard candy as an alternative to eating. If he says it's O.K., make sure the patient's aware he must not swallow the candy.
• Give the patient and his family emotional support. Emphasize the positive aspects of his condition. Encourage his family to find ways to cheer him.

Hyperalimentation therapy complications: What to do

If your patient's getting hyperalimentation therapy through a central line, do your best to prevent complications by observing strict aseptic technique, and providing meticulous site care at all times.

Remember, however, that complications can arise no matter how careful you are. To discover how to cope with them, read the following chart.

Your observations	Possible problems
Redness and swelling at catheter site	• Early infection • Phlebitis
Drainage at site	• Infection • Catheter-caused injury to the thoracic duct, causing chylothorax
Edema at catheter site	• Extravasation from dislodged catheter
Moist dressing	• Catheter has become dislodged, causing I.V. fluid to leak onto dressing
Skin ulcerations	• Excessive sweating under bandage • Sensitivity to iodine or elastic
Labored breathing, respiratory collapse	• Air embolism caused when disconnected tubing has allowed air to become trapped in the circulatory system • Hydrothorax
Engorged neck veins, moist respirations, elevated blood pressure	• Pulmonary edema from fluid overload • Congestive heart failure

COMPLICATIONS

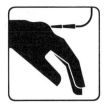

Nursing considerations

• Notify the doctor. He may discontinue therapy. Culture the hyperalimentation solution bottle, tubing, and at least 4" of the catheter.

• Notify the doctor. He'll probably remove the catheter, place the patient in a high Fowler's position, and apply firm digital pressure to the insertion site for 5 to 10 minutes. Culture the bottle, tubing, and catheter.

• Lower the solution container, pinch the tubing and flashbulb, and check for blood backflow. If no blood backflow appears, call the doctor.

• Undress and check all connections and site. If tubing's loose, tighten it. If the insertion site has become enlarged, the doctor may order a pressure dressing applied to stop the oozing.

• Redress the site without applying benzoin or Betadine. Instead, clean the site thoroughly, but gently with soap and sterile water. Let it dry. Then, cover the entire area with a sterile gauze pad. Tape the pad in place with nonallergenic tape. Take care not to place tape on the affected areas.

• Place patient in Trendelenburg position, lying on his left side. This position will send air into the heart's right side, where it can be absorbed. Call doctor.

• Place the patient in a high Fowler's position. Administer oxygen and monitor his vital signs. Set the flow rate to keep the vein patent. Call the doctor.

Changing the tubing

1 *When a patient's receiving hyperalimentation, you should change the tubing at least every 48 hours, as recommended by the Center for Disease Control (CDC).*

To do this properly, follow the instructions below. Make sure you use aseptic technique throughout the procedure. (Your hospital may also require you to wear sterile gloves.)

Place a 2" x 2" sterile gauze pad under the catheter connection to create a sterile field. Check the connection. If it's very snug, use a hemostat to loosen it before you try to disconnect the tube entirely. *Note:* Be careful you don't apply too much pressure or you'll crack the hub. If you do, notify the doctor. He'll decide whether or not the catheter should be replaced.

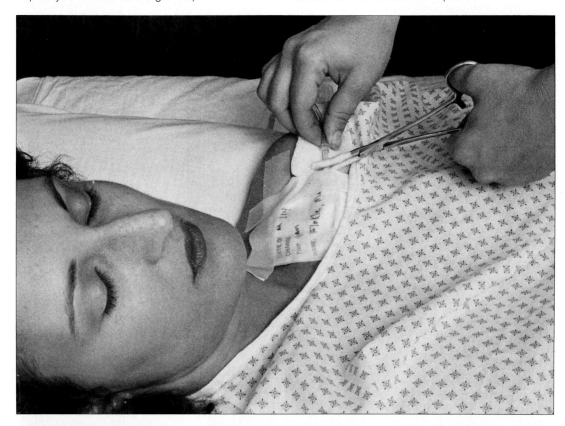

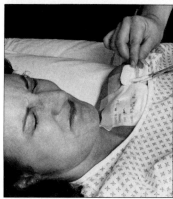

2 Instruct your patient to lie flat. Ask her to perform the Valsalva maneuver (closing her mouth and bearing down). This will create internal pressure, making an air embolism less likely.

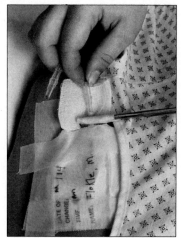

3 Now, quickly rotate the used intravenous tube until it detaches from the hub. Discard it.

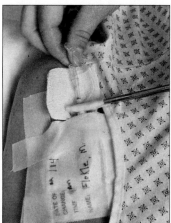

4 Then, insert the new primed tubing into the hub, making sure it's secure. Encourage the patient to relax. Document what you've done.

Hyperalimentation

Changing the dressing

1 *To properly care for the patient receiving hyperalimentation, you'll have to change the dressing on her insertion site at least three times weekly, or immediately, if it becomes loose or wet. To find out how, read this photostory carefully.*

Before you begin, explain to your patient exactly what you're about to do. Maintain strict aseptic technique throughout the procedure, beginning with a thorough hand washing.

Does the hospital require you and the patient to wear face masks during the dressing change? Explain why masks are necessary, to keep her hyperalimentation site uncontaminated. Then, slip your mask on, and place the other loosely over the patient's mouth. However, *never* put a mask on a patient who needs oxygen or who has a nasogastric tube in place.

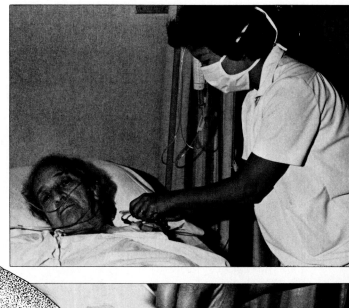

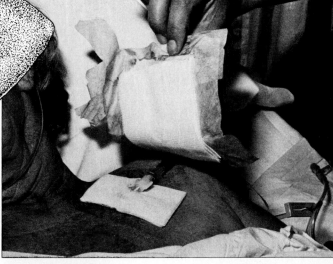

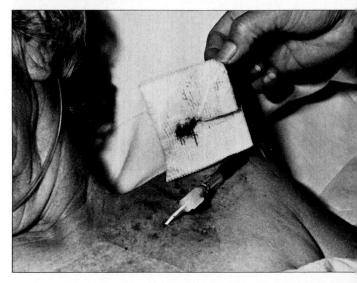

2 Next, place the patient in a supine position. Turn her head away from the dressing to make the insertion site more accessible and to minimize the risk of contamination.

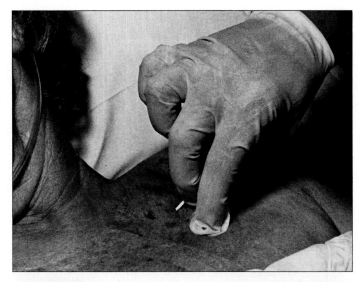

5 Put on sterile gloves, and clean around the insertion site with acetone. Work in a circular motion, from the site outward. As you do, take care not to jostle the catheter, or you'll increase the chance of infection.
    Caution: Remember, acetone will have a corrosive effect on the catheter. If they come in contact, immediately wash the catheter with a saline solution.

3 Remove the old dressing, taking care not to disturb the catheter. As you do, pinch the soiled surfaces together so they don't contaminate your hands.
    🖎 *Nursing tip:* If your dressing kit has no plastic disposal bag for the discarded dressing, make sure a wastebasket's nearby before you begin the procedure.

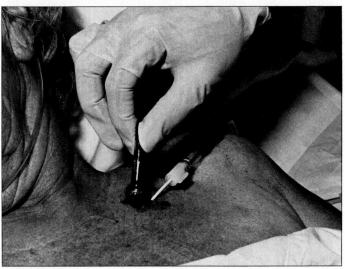

6 Now, clean the site with povidine-iodine, using the circular motion already described. Let the povidine-iodine dry naturally. Don't fan your hands over the site. Doing so will only increase the risk of contamination.

4 Now, examine the site for any signs of infection; for example, discharge, inflammation, or soreness. If you suspect infection, culture the drainage, send the labeled specimen to the lab with a requisition slip, and notify the doctor. Then, check the catheter to make sure it's positioned correctly.

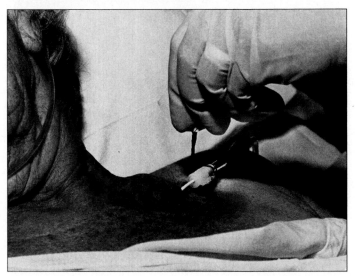

7 Apply antimicrobial ointment to the insertion site. If the catheter was taped in place, check the tape to make sure it's clean. Remove soiled tape and replace it with sterile tape, using the chevron taping method described on page 37. Then, remove all soiled dressings from the patient's room.
    For complete details on how to tape a hyperalimentation catheter using other methods, see pages 33 and 36.

Hyperalimentation

How to remove a central line

1 *At the end of hyperali-mentation therapy, the doctor will order the central line removed. Nursing responsibilities vary among hospitals. If removal of central lines is a nursing responsibility at your hospital, here's what to do.*

[Inset] First, wash your hands, and assemble the equipment shown in this photo: acetone, sterile gauze pads, tape, forceps, **scissors, and sterile gloves.**

[Illustration] Explain to the patient what you're about to do. Then, loosen the tape on the dressing and remove the dressing, taking care not to contaminate your hands. You can use acetone to remove tape marks from the patient's skin, but be careful not to contaminate the site.

Then, put on a pair of sterile gloves. Remove the sutures securing the catheter, as shown in this illustration. *Important:* Take care to avoid cutting the catheter when you remove the sutures.

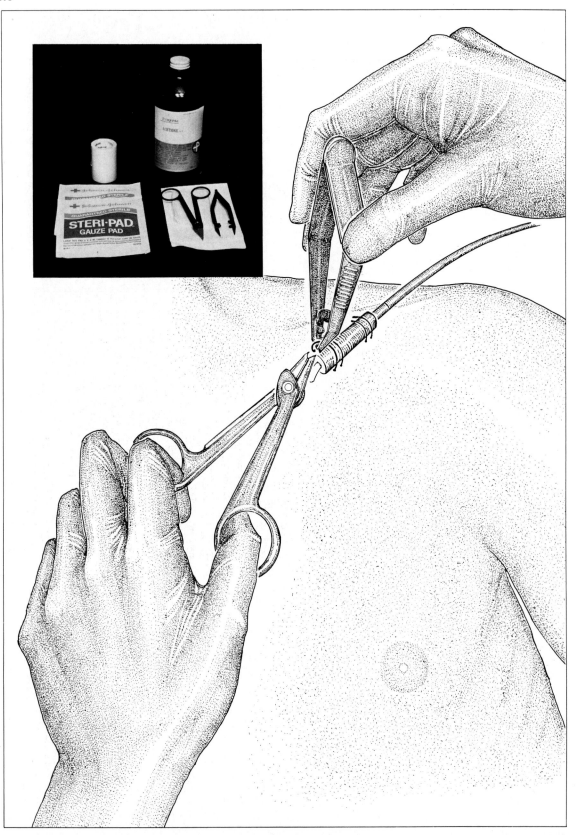

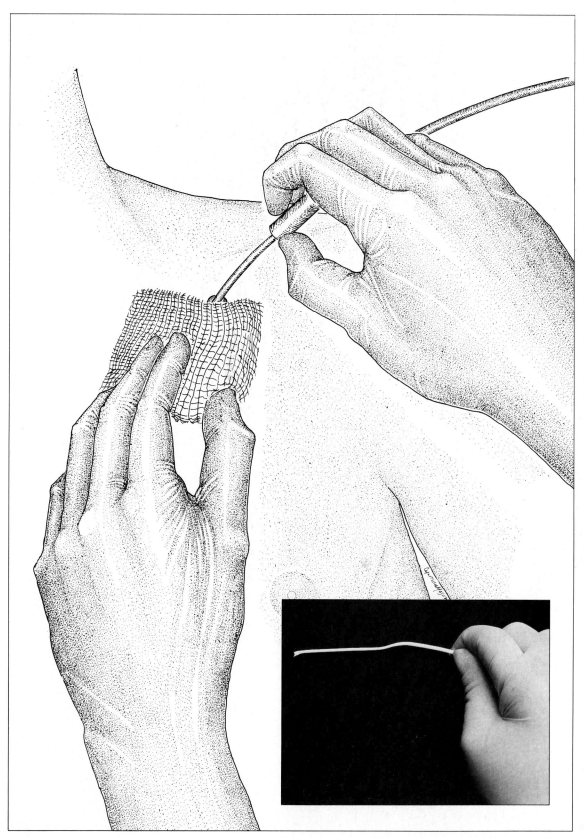

2 Now, working slowly and carefully, withdraw the catheter from the vein, as shown in this illustration. Using a 2" x 2" sterile gauze pad, apply manual pressure over the site for 1 minute. *Note:* If the catheter's in a leg vein, apply manual pressure for at least 5 minutes.

[Inset] Inspect the catheter closely. If it's ragged or damaged, notify the doctor immediately. A catheter embolism may be present. Since a damaged catheter also may trigger an infection, have the catheter tip cultured, as recommended by the Center for Disease Control (CDC). To do this, cut off 1" or 2" of the catheter tip with sterile scissors. Put it in a sterile test tube or container, and send it to the lab for analysis.

Examine the insertion site for signs of infection. If you suspect it, culture any drainage from the wound.

Then, apply antimicrobial ointment, and tape down a pressure bandage.

Document what you've done in your nurses' notes and in the patient's care plan. Include the date and time, the catheter's condition (at the time of removal), and the condition of the insertion site. Also note the type of dressing and ointment applied. If you sent the catheter tip or drainage specimen to the lab for culture, include that information too.

After 1 hour, remove the pressure bandage and dressing, and apply more antimicrobial ointment. Cover the site with an adhesive bandage strip.

I.V. fat emulsions

What if hyperalimentation's not sufficient to maintain your patient's weight and growth rate? The doctor will probably order a fat emulsion. Do you know:
• When a fat emulsion should or shouldn't be given?
• How it's administered?
• What complications it can cause?
• How to minimize these complications?
    The following pages will answer these questions and more. Read them so you can effectively manage the patient on this type of therapy.

INDICATIONS/CONTRAINDICATIONS

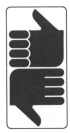

I.V. fat emulsions: Who gets them?

You'll probably be giving I.V. fat emulsion to your patient if he:
• Needs calories and can't tolerate the high percentage of dextrose contained in hyperalimentation solutions
• Needs protein and nitrogen supplements; for example, a patient with cancer, stenosis, or a peptic ulcer
• Needs more essential fatty acids than contained in hyperalimentation solutions
• Needs general nutritional improvement; particularly the preoperative patient.

Don't give an I.V. fat emulsion to the patient who:
• Suffers from a disturbance of normal fat metabolism, such as, hyperlipemia
• Suffers from severe hepatic disease. Remember, the liver helps utilize fatty acids.
• Has a blood coagulation defect caused by a decreased blood-platelet count
• Has a pulmonary disease. Remember, I.V. fat emulsion goes to the heart first and could affect it adversely.
• Suffers from lipoid nephrosis
• Suffers from hepatocellular damage
• Has bone marrow dyscrasia
• Is being treated with anabolic inhibitory drugs.

Gathering your equipment

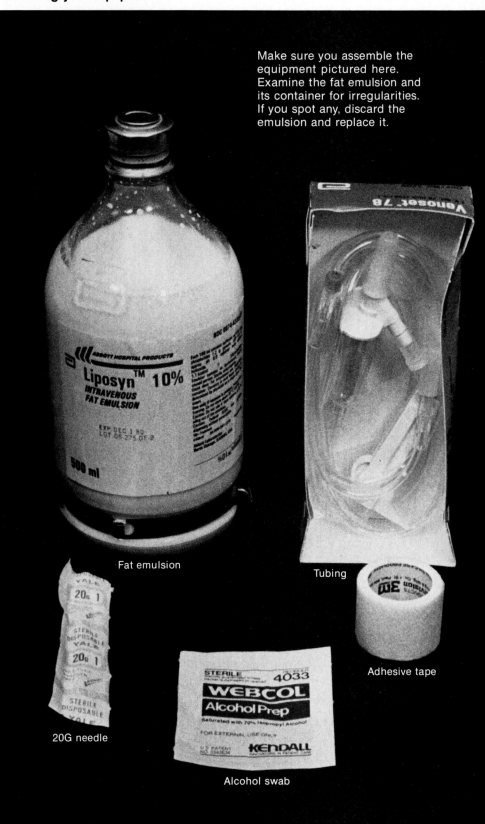

Make sure you assemble the equipment pictured here. Examine the fat emulsion and its container for irregularities. If you spot any, discard the emulsion and replace it.

Fat emulsion

Tubing

20G needle

Alcohol swab

Adhesive tape

Administering a fat emulsion

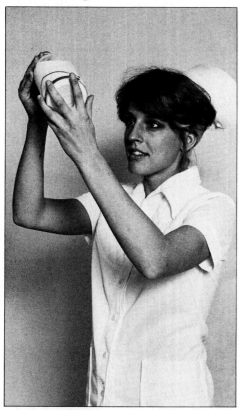

1 *What's involved in administering an I.V. fat emulsion? Begin by making sure it's been stored between 39° and 46° F. (4° and 8° C.). Then, let it stand for 30 minutes at room temperature before using it.*

Examine it for signs of instability, as the nurse is doing in this photo. Are there any inconsistencies in texture or color? If there are, discard it.

If the emulsion's O.K., remove the cap from the container and swab the stopper with alcohol. *Important:* Never shake or add any fluid to a container of fat emulsion. If you do, you'll ruin the emulsion.

2 Now, spike the container.

☟ *Nursing tip:* To prevent the spike from disconnecting, you may want to tape it to the container. When you do, however, avoid placing stress on the tubing.

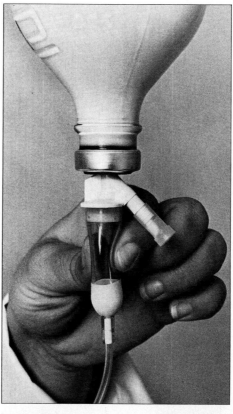

3 Now, clamp the tubing closed, and squeeze the drip chamber until it's half full of solution.

☟ *Nursing tip:* Have a clamp handy in case the tubing clamp breaks.

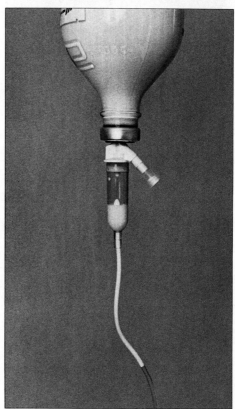

4 Open the clamp slightly, and slowly prime the tubing. If you prime too fast, you'll cause air bubbles to form in the tubing.

Close the clamp.

I.V. fat emulsions

Administering a fat emulsion continued

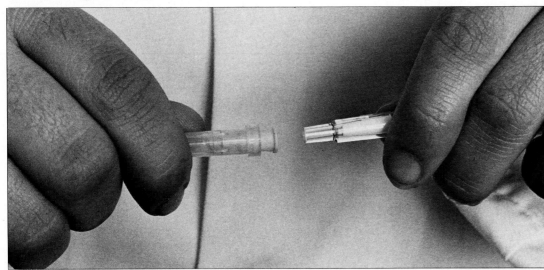

5 Attach a 20G 1'' needle to the end of the fat emulsion line. Now you're ready to hang the container. Remember, you must always hang a fat emulsion container higher than the hyperalimentation solution bottle. Otherwise, the fat emulsion, being more viscous, may back up into the primary line.

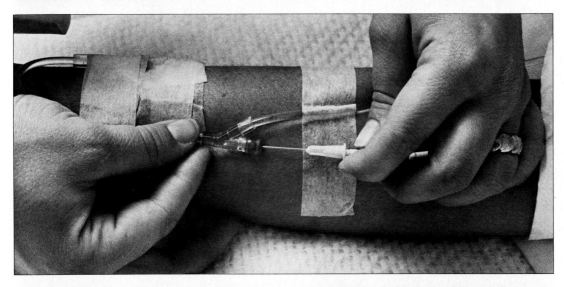

6 Swab the secondary port on the primary line with alcohol. (Using the secondary port minimizes the mixing time of the emulsion and the hyperalimentation solution before they enter the bloodstream.)
Now, insert the needle into the port. *Important:* Make sure there's no filter below the secondary port. Fat emulsion particles, which are 0.5 micron in size, won't pass through a filter.

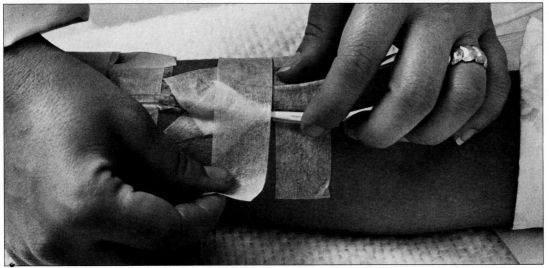

7 Next, loop the tubing, and securely tape the needle and adapter to the primary line, as shown in this photo.

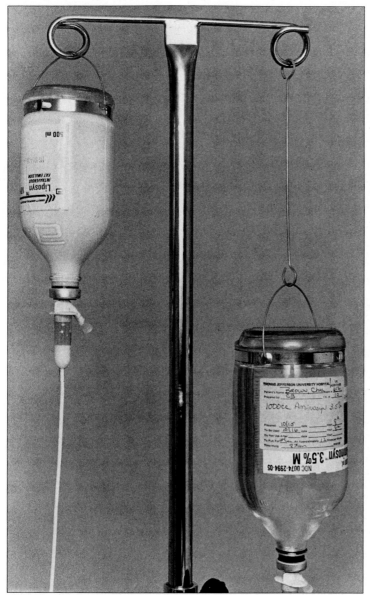

8 Open the roller clamp, and begin feeding the fat emulsion at the recommended rate. For the first 30 minutes, deliver 1 ml per minute. If no complications develop, increase the dosage to as much as 500 ml every 4 hours. Don't exceed a daily dose of 2.5 grams of emulsion per Kg of patient's body weight. (For information about complications that can develop from I.V. fat emulsion therapy, see box at right.)

📠 *Nursing tip:* If possible, restrict I.V. fat emulsion infusions to daytime hours, using nightly breaks to simulate a normal eating pattern. This pattern will allow the patient to rest during the night and also helps diminish his nocturnal urinary flow.

When the infusion's completed and you've disconnected the container, discard it. Don't use any fat emulsion that remains.

If you must hang another container of fat emulsion, replace the tubing, but leave the original needle. If you're not hanging another bottle, remove the entire set (bottle, tubing, and needle), and discard it.

Caring for the patient receiving I.V. fat emulsion

Carefully explain the purpose of I.V. fat emulsion therapy to the patient, and answer any questions he has.

• Once the I.V. line has been established, use an electronic control device to maintain an even flow rate. By doing this, you'll avoid giving the patient a fatty-acid overload.

• Regularly measure the patient's fluid intake and output, caloric intake, and temperature. Take daily blood studies to determine the level of free-floating triglycerides. Document your findings.

• If the patient's being given I.V. fat emulsion over a long time, monitor his ability to eliminate the infused fat. Perform hepatic function tests. If his liver function's impaired, inform the doctor.

---COMPLICATIONS---

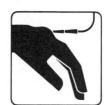

**Adverse reactions to
I.V. fat emulsion therapy**

Immediate reactions (up to 2½ hours)
Temperature rise
Flushing
Sweating
Pressure sensations over eyes
Nausea, vomiting, headache
Chest and back pains
Dyspnea, cyanosis

Delayed reactions (within 10 days)
Hepatomegaly
Splenomegaly
Thrombocytopenia
Focal seizures
Hyperlipemia
Hepatic damage
Jaundice
Hemorrhagic diathesis
Gastroduodenal ulcer

If the patient experiences any of these reactions after fat emulsion therapy, notify the doctor.

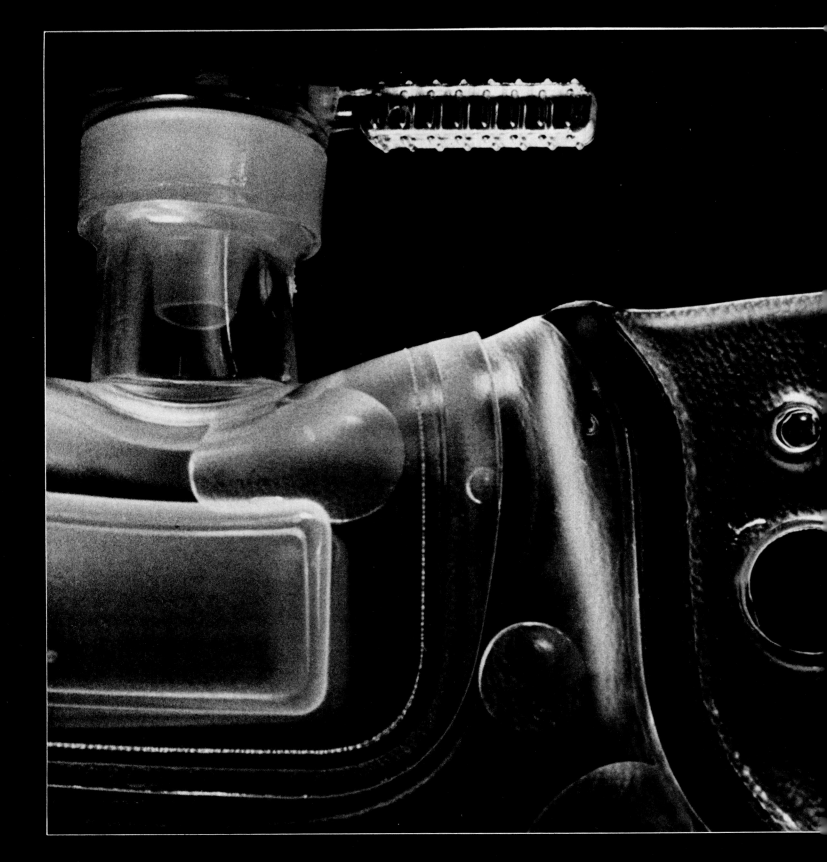

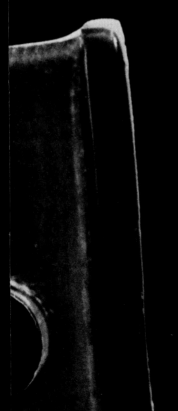

Administering Whole Blood and Its Components

Blood transfusions

Phlebotomy

Blood transfusions

You may see blood being transfused everyday and think it's a simple matter. But don't be misled. Blood transfusion's a very complex procedure. The patient's health depends, in large part, on your knowledge and ability. You should know:
• the difference between administration sets.
• how to use special accessory equipment.
• why the doctor may choose a blood component rather than whole blood.
• what complications may arise from a transfusion, and how to treat them.

If you're not familiar with these specifics, read the following pages carefully.

What blood does

As you know, blood plays a fundamental role in maintaining the body. It carries everything the tissues require for energy or synthesis, and removes all cellular waste products. Blood functions by:
• supplying oxygen and nutrients for tissue maintenance, growth, and repair.
• transporting cellular waste, including carbon dioxide, to the elimination organs.
• providing a defense against infection by transporting antibodies.
• regulating and equalizing body temperature.
• helping to maintain the tissues' acid-base balance.
• regulating the tissues' water and electrolyte content.

Because blood has so many important functions, any deficiency in it requires correction. To learn which blood components are needed to correct certain deficiencies, read on.

Blood: A microscopic view

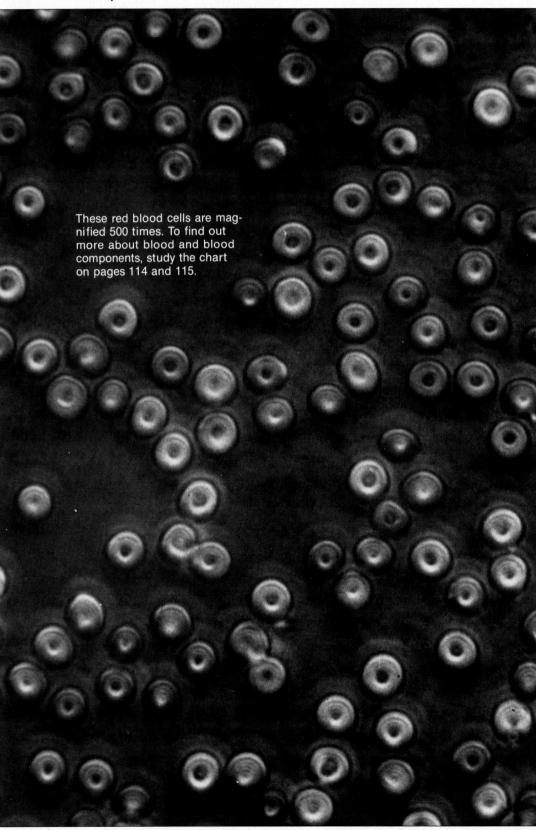

These red blood cells are magnified 500 times. To find out more about blood and blood components, study the chart on pages 114 and 115.

Preventing transfusion hazards

You can minimize the hazards of blood transfusion by taking great care to avoid mistakes. Proper identifying and matching procedures are crucial. Read what follows to learn how they're done.

Fill out the requisition form with care, using the sample printed below as a guide. Make sure you complete the form. Otherwise, the blood bank won't process it and you'll waste precious time.

Before you draw a blood sample, make sure you have the right patient. Don't just check his chart. Ask him for his full name, as you explain the importance of accuracy to him. Refer to his wristband for confirmation. Carefully check and record all the data written on it. If you must draw a blood sample from an unidentified emergency patient, make sure he's been assigned a temporary identifying number. Now, send the blood sample to the lab so it can be typed and crossmatched.

When you go to the blood bank to pick up blood for your patient, take along a copy of the requisition form. As the blood bank technologist gives you the unit of blood, match the name and room number on the blood bag label with the name and room number on your requisition form. Then, match the hospital number, the ABO group and Rh type, the unit number, the blood donor number, and the expiration date.

If everything checks out, bring the blood back to the patient's bedside. You'll find the lab report prepared from the blood sample you took attached to the blood bag. With another nurse assisting to insure accuracy, match the patient to the blood before beginning the transfusion. Compare the information on the lab's blood type record with:
• the patient's name and identification number
• the number on the blood bag label
• the ABO group and Rh type on the blood bag label.

If all these factors match up, sign the lab's blood type record, and begin the transfusion. If these factors don't match up, contact the doctor immediately. Don't begin the transfusion until you've resolved the discrepancies.

Remember to document the entire procedure after you've started the transfusion.

Blood typing and crossmatching

Compatibility's a critical concern in blood transfusion. If the blood you infuse doesn't match the patient's blood, the results can be fatal. To insure accuracy, a laboratory technologist runs tests on the blood sample to determine the patient's blood type (A, B, AB, or O) and whether the blood is Rh positive or Rh negative.

Blood types are differentiated by their agglutinogen (an antigen) and agglutinin (an antibody) content. Agglutinogen is found in the red cells and agglutinin is found in the plasma or serum. Study this chart to see how the types differ:

Blood type	Agglutinogen type	Agglutinin type
A	A	anti-B
B	B	anti-A
AB	A and B	none
O	none	anti-A and anti-B

Rh typing determines whether or not the red cells in the sample blood contain the Rh factor. Blood with the Rh factor (common to the majority of people in the United States) is called Rh positive. Blood lacking it is called Rh negative.

Mixing the wrong types of blood is prevented by crossmatching. After the lab technologist types the patient's blood, he'll crossmatch it with the blood to be infused. Crossmatching tells whether or not the patient's blood is compatible with the blood he's going to receive.

Each year, doctors learn more about blood complexities and the importance of precise crossmatching. To guard your patient's health, never mix blood or Rh types unless the doctor orders it in an emergency. In such a situation, you may be ordered to deliver the following: types A, B, or AB blood for a patient with AB type blood; or type O blood for a patient with A, B, or AB blood. The doctor may also consider giving Rh negative blood to a patient typed Rh positive.

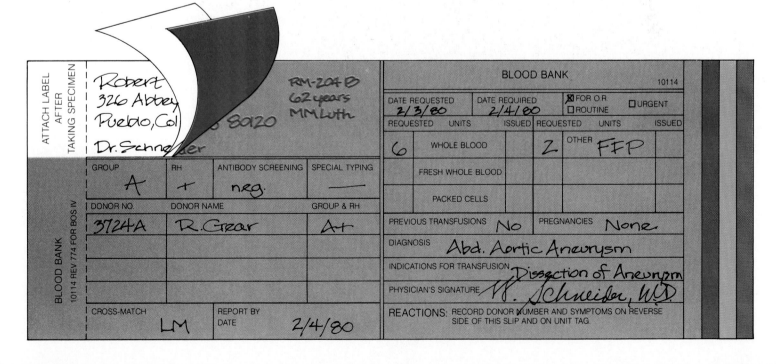

Blood transfusions

Nurses' guide to whole blood and its components

Blood can be broken down into a variety of components. Each component treats a particular blood deficiency, and each component has qualities all its own. How can you keep them all straight? This chart will help. You might want to copy it and keep it nearby for handy reference.

Type	Description	Indications	Contraindications	
Whole blood	Complete, unadulterated blood	• To restore an adequate volume of blood in hemorrhaging, trauma, or burn patients	• When the patient doesn't need volume increase and a specific component is available	
Red blood cells (packed, frozen)	Whole blood with 80% of the supernatant plasma removed	• To correct red blood cell deficiency and improve oxygen-carrying capacity of blood • To transfuse organ transplant patients or for patients with repeated febrile transfusion reactions, use frozen-thawed RBCs because the allogeneic leukocytes are destroyed with freezing.	• When the patient's anemic from a deficiency of the hematopoietic nutrients; for example, iron, vitamin B$_{12}$, or folic acid • When the patient's asymptomatic, but you must raise his hematocrit level	
White blood cells (leukocyte concentrate)	Whole blood with all the red blood cells and 80% of the supernatant plasma removed	• To treat the patient who has life-threatening granulocytopenia from intensive chemotherapy, especially if his infections aren't responsive to antibiotics	• When the patient's health depends on the recovery of his bone marrow functions	
Plasma (fresh, fresh frozen)	Uncoagulated plasma separated from whole blood	• To treat a clotting factor deficiency (when specific concentrates are unavailable or precise deficiency's unknown), hypovolemia, or a patient with a severe hepatic disease who has a limited synthesis of plasma coagulation factors • To prevent dilutional hypocoagulability	• When blood coagulation can be corrected with available specific therapy • When patient needs only albumin	
Platelets	Platelet sediment from platelet-rich plasma, resuspended in 30 to 50 ml of plasma	• To treat the patient with thrombocytopenia whose bleeding is caused by the following: decreased platelet production, increased platelet destruction, functionally abnormal platelets, or massive transfusions of stored blood (dilutional thrombocytopenia)	• When bleeding's unrelated to decreased number of platelets or abnormal function of platelets • When the patient's suffering from post-transfusion purpura or thrombotic thrombocytopenic purpura	
Plasma protein fraction	5% solution of selected proteins from pooled plasma in a buffered, stabilized saline diluent	• To treat hypovolemic shock or hypoproteinemia. • For initial treatment of infants in shock or children who are dehydrated or who have electrolyte deficiencies • May be used cautiously when the patient has congestive heart failure from added fluid and salt load; or has renal or hepatic failure from added protein load.	• When the patient has a clotting factor deficiency	
Albumin 5% (buffered saline) **Albumin 25%** (salt-poor)	Heat-treated, aqueous, chemically processed fraction of pooled plasma	• To treat shock from burns, trauma, surgery, or infections • To prevent marked hemoconcentration • To maintain appropriate electrolyte balance • To treat hypoproteinemia (with or without edema)	• When the patient has severe anemia or cardiac failure	
Factor VIII (cryoprecipitate concentrate AHF)	Cold-insoluble portion of plasma recovered from fresh frozen plasma	• To treat a patient with hemophilia A • To control bleeding associated with Factor VIII deficiency • To replace fibrinogen or Factor XIII	• When the patient has undefined coagulation defects	
Factors II, VII, IX, X Complex	Lyophilized, commercially prepared solution drawn from pooled plasma	• Prior to surgery to treat congenital deficiencies of Factors II, VII, IX, or X Complex and provide a hemostatic level • To arrest severe hemorrhaging	• When the patient has hepatic disease that has caused fibrinolysis • When the patient has intravascular coagulation and is not undergoing heparin therapy	

Cross-matching	Shelf life	Administration techniques	Special considerations
Necessary	21 days at 41° F. (5° C.)	• Administer by straight line set, Y-set, or microaggregate recipient set.	• Although whole blood is seldom transfused, components that are necessary—and frequently administered—are extracted from it. • Plasma protein fraction or albumin are given as volume expanders while tests are run to determine the patient's exact component needs.
Necessary	For stored fresh packed cells, 21 days; or 24 hours after opening For stored frozen cells, 3 years; or 24 hours after thawing	• Administer by straight line set, Y-set, or microaggregate recipient set.	• Red blood cells have the same oxygen-carrying capacity as whole blood without the hazards of overload. Their use avoids the buildup of potassium and ammonia that sometimes occurs in the plasma of stored blood. Frozen-thawed RBCs are extremely expensive.
Must be ABO compatible (preferably HLA compatible) [human leukocyte group A antigen])	24 hours after collection at 41° F. (5° C.)	• Administer by any straight line set. • Use with standard in-line blood filter. • Dosage: 1 unit daily until infection clears (usually within 5 days)	Important: WBC infusion induces a fever and can cause mild hypertension, severe chills, disorientation, and hallucinations. Try to control the patient's chills with antipyretics or blankets. Then, treat the hypertension, if necessary.
Unnecessary	For fresh plasma, within 6 hours after collection For fresh, frozen plasma, 12 months at −4° F. (−18° C.); or 2 hours after thawing	• Administer as rapidly as possible by any straight line set.	• Normal saline solution not needed for Y-set, because the component contains no RBCs.
Unnecessary (donor plasma and recipient's RBCs should be ABO compatible)	Up to 72 hours after whole blood collection	• Administer as rapidly as possible (uninterrupted) by syringe or component drip set only. • Don't use a standard in-line blood filter. Instead, use a non-wettable filter. • Dosage: 2 units per Kg of body weight to raise the platelet count by at least 50,000/cu mm	• Usually administered when patient's platelet count drops below 10,000/cu mm • For the patient with a history of side effects: administer antihistamines before platelet transfusion. Slower administration may be necessary to prevent overload. • Least hazardous when given fresh • Must be constantly agitated during storage
Unnecessary	5 years if refrigerated; 3 years at room temperature	• Administer by any straight line set at a rate and volume dependent on the patient's condition and response.	• Should not be mixed in the same line with protein hydrolysates and alcohol solutions • Often given as a volume expander in place of whole blood while crossmatching is being completed
Unnecessary	5 years at 35.6° F. (2° C.); 3 years at room temperature	• Administer by provided set undiluted, or diluted with saline solution or 5% dextrose in water. • For a patient with normal blood volume or hypoproteinemia: administer slowly (1 ml/min) to prevent rapid plasma volume expansion. • For a patient in shock: administer as rapidly as possible.	• Can't transmit hepatitis because it's heat-treated at 140° F. (60° C.) for 10 hours • Often given as a volume expander in place of whole blood while crossmatching is being completed
Unnecessary (donor plasma and recipient's RBCs should be ABO compatible)	12 months, if frozen at −4° F. (−18° C.); up to 6 hours after thawing	• Administer as rapidly as possible by syringe or component drip set only. • Initial dose: 2 units per/12 Kg of body weight. After that, 1 unit per/12 Kg of body weight	• Risk of hepatitis same as with whole blood
Unnecessary	Refer to manufacturer's expiration date	• Administer by any straight line set. • Dosage: based on desired level and patient's body weight	• Very high hepatitis risk

Blood transfusions

How to use a straight-line blood set

1 *The straight-line blood set is the most common blood administration set. Here's how to use it correctly:*

Begin by examining the line pictured here. Note that the filter's *inside* the drip chamber. Now, move the roller clamp so it's directly under the drip chamber, or as near to it as possible. Then close it. Remove the protective cap from the spike.

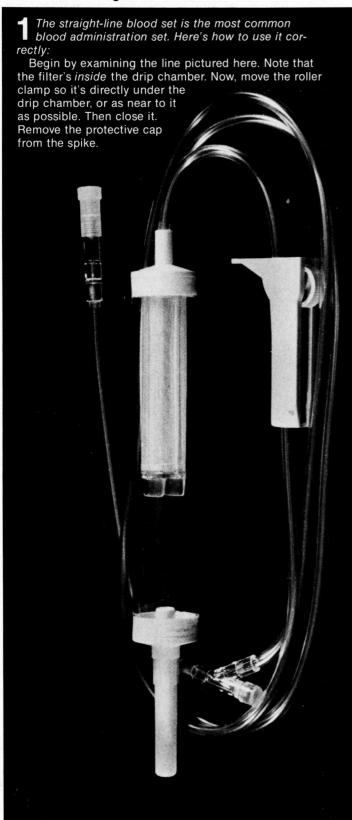

2 Now you're ready to expose the port at the top of the blood bag. To do so, pull back the tabs, as shown here. *Important:* Don't touch the port, because doing so could contaminate it.

Are you giving whole blood? If you are, remember that red cells usually settle on the bottom and plasma tends to rise. Always mix whole blood thoroughly before you administer it. Rocking the bag from side to side during administration helps keep it mixed, but don't shake it too vigorously, or you'll cause cell destruction.

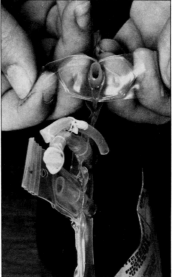

3 Next, insert the spike into the port with a twisting motion, but take special care not to pierce the bag with the spike. If that happened, you'd have to discard and replace the bag. Hang the set.

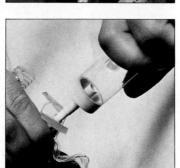

4 If you're using a set with a separate filter and drip chamber, fill the filter with blood by squeezing the drip chamber. But, don't squeeze the filter or you'll rupture it.

Does the set you're using have a combination drip chamber/filter, as shown here? Fill this type chamber by squeezing it directly.

With either set, make sure the filter's completely immersed in blood before proceeding. Then, open the roller clamp and prime the tubing, taking care to expel all the air. Tap the filter to dislodge any trapped air bubbles.

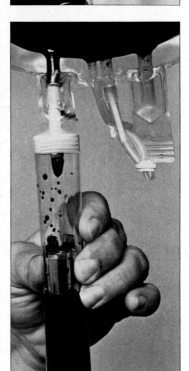

5 Now, you're ready to connect the blood set. Perform a venipuncture, using a 19G (or larger) ONC or INC, following the procedure on pages 38 to 42. Suppose the patient already has an I.V. line in place. First, make sure the I.V. needle is 19G or larger. If it isn't, replace it. A smaller gauge needle will clog if you use it to deliver blood.

If the needle *can* accommodate blood, follow these steps to connect the straight-line blood set to the primary line.

First, attach a 16G or 18G needle to the adapter on the blood line. Uncap the needle, and prime the blood line to remove any trapped air. Recap the needle.

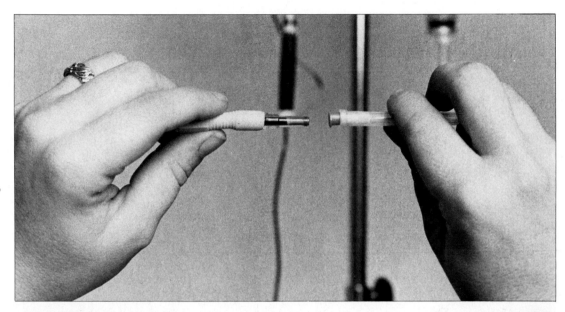

6 Now, check the primary solution. If it isn't a normal saline solution, close the roller clamp, unhook the container, and remove the spike. You can cap this container for later use, or discard it. But in either case, document the amount of solution absorbed on the patient's intake/output record.

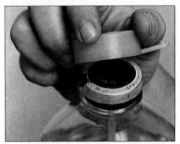

7 Using the original tubing, spike a container of normal saline solution and hang it. Open the roller clamp to flush the line.

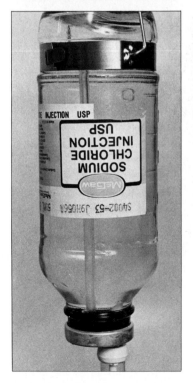

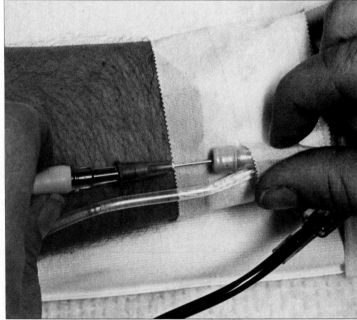

8 Insert the blood line's needle into the secondary port on the primary I.V. line. Open the blood line clamp, and adjust the flow rate. Remember to clamp the line to the saline solution.

If the blood line clamp's completely open and the flow rate's inadequate, consider the following: the size of the catheter may be too small to administer blood; the blood may be infiltrating into the subcutaneous tissue; or the vein may be inadequate. Correct these conditions.

Suppose none of these conditions apply. Try raising the I.V. pole to extend the distance between the blood unit and the insertion site. (This will increase the gravitational pull on the blood.) If this doesn't help—and you're using packed blood cells—open the roller clamp on the saline solution line slightly to dilute the concentrated blood.

Blood transfusions

Using a microaggregate recipient set

1 *When should you use a microaggregate recipient set? Whenever you want to deliver large amounts of stored whole
blood or packed cells. As you may know, red blood cells gradu-
ally deteriorate in storage. These destroyed cells are called
microaggregates. Examine the set in this photo. It features a
special filter that prevents these microaggregates from entering
and clogging your patient's circulatory system. In addition,
the tubing has a larger lumen, which allows the blood to be delivered more rapidly. Here's how to use it:*
    Begin the procedure by making sure the roller clamp's closed.

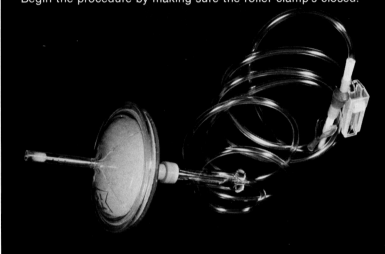

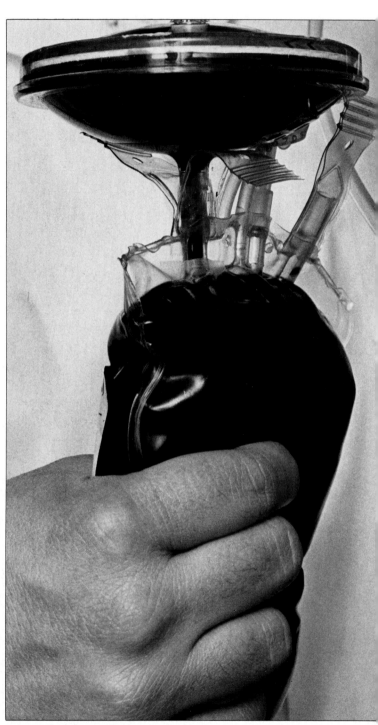

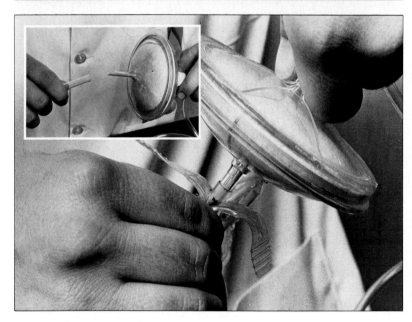

2 [Inset] Remove the spike cover. Then,
expose the port at the top of the blood
bag. To do this, pull back the tabs.
Important: Don't touch the port, because
you'll contaminate it.
    Now, insert the spike into the blood bag
port with a twisting motion, as shown here.

3 Invert the blood bag, and open the
roller clamp. Gently compress the
blood bag until the filter's completely full.

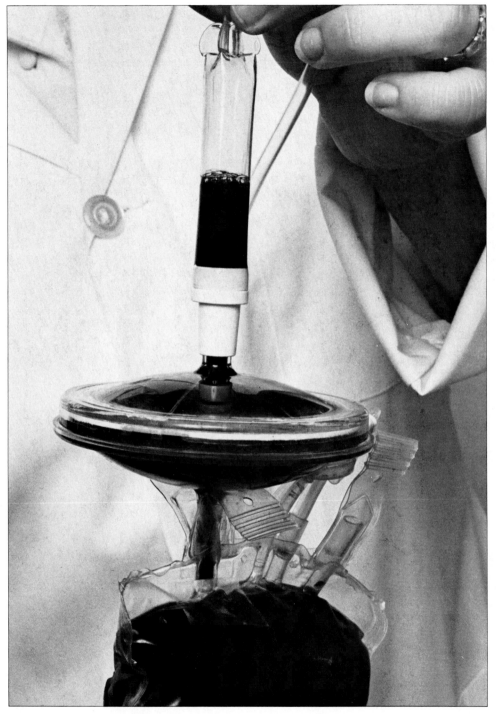

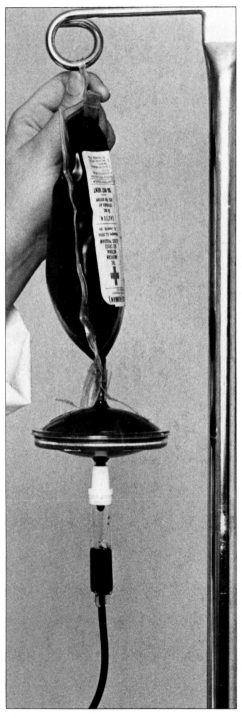

4 Continue to compress the blood bag until the drip chamber's half full. If the bag won't squeeze readily, loosen the needle adapter cover and try again. Invert the bag to help expel air from the tubing. Gently tap the filter a few times to dislodge any trapped air bubbles.

5 Next, close the clamp, and hang the blood bag on an I.V. pole, as shown here. Open the clamp, and prime the tubing and needle. Now you're ready to start transfusing the blood. To connect the set to your patient correctly, follow the same steps outlined for the straight-line blood set, on page 116.

Blood transfusions

Using a Y-set

1 *When do you need a Y-set for a transfusion? Consider these instances: Suppose you're ordered to transfuse packed cells. Because of the component's viscosity, you may need to run saline solution with it to dilute it. Or suppose you're going to attach the blood line to a primary I.V. line. You'll have to flush the primary line first with normal saline solution. In either case, you'll need a Y-set. The following photostory will show you how to use it.*

Here's what the set looks like. Before you begin the procedure, make sure you close all clamps on the Y-set: the main flow rate clamp, the clamp on the saline solution line (with the vented tubing), and the clamp on the blood line (with the unvented tubing).

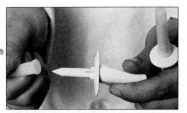

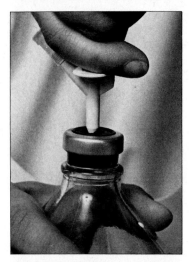

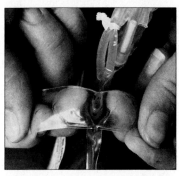

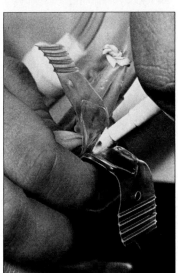

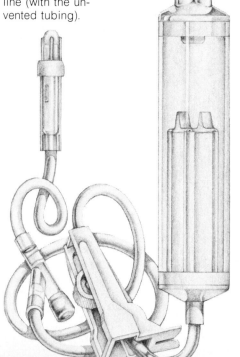

2 Now, remove the cap from the spike on the saline solution line.

3 Swab the port of the saline solution container with alcohol. Then insert the spike into the container, as shown in this photo.
Important: Never use anything but normal saline solution with whole blood or its components. The use of any other fluid causes hemolysis.

4 Next, remove the cap from the blood line spike. Then, expose the blood bag's port by pulling back the two tabs at the top of the bag. *Important:* Don't touch the port, because you'll contaminate it.

5 Insert the blood line spike into the blood bag port.

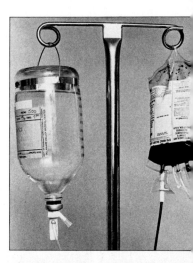

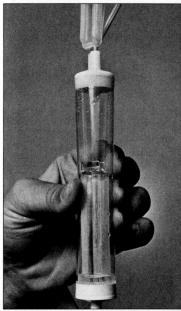

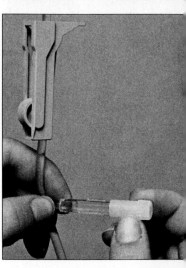

6 Then, hang the entire Y-set on an I.V. pole, as shown here.

Important: Change the Y-set tubing every 4 hours.

7 Open the saline solution line clamp. Squeeze the combination drip chamber/filter until it's half full.

8 Remove the needle adapter cover. Open the main flow rate clamp. Prime the tubing. Then, close these clamps, and recap the needle adapter.

If the patient has no I.V. line in place, perform venipuncture, as described on page 31. If he already has an I.V. line, proceed as follows.

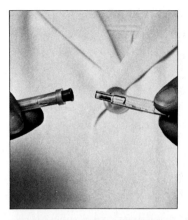

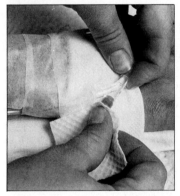

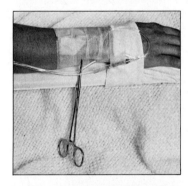

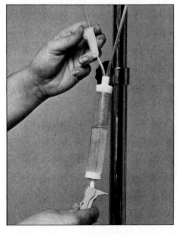

9 Remove the needle adapter cover. Attach a 16G or 18G needle to the adapter and prime the line.

10 With alcohol, swab the injection port nearest to the insertion site.

11 Then, close the primary line clamp. To prevent blood backup into the primary line, use a hemostat to clamp the primary line just above the injection port. Next, insert the needle into the injection port.

12 Open the saline solution clamp and the main flow rate clamp to flush the entire line with saline solution. Then, close both clamps. Make sure there's no in-line filter between the injection port and the insertion site on the primary line. Filters on primary lines will clog when used with blood.

13 Open the blood line clamp. Squeeze the combination drip chamber/filter on the Y-set until the filter's completely immersed in blood.

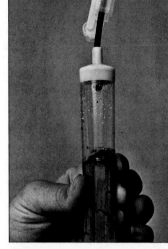

14 Open the Y-set's main clamp, and adjust the blood's flow rate. Keep the primary line clamped off, as this photo shows, so the blood doesn't back up into the tubing. Document the entire procedure, as explained on page 43.

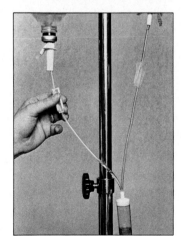

15 When the blood bag is empty, close the blood line clamp. Open the saline solution clamp to flush the tubing with saline solution. Then, close the remaining clamps.

16 To start the primary I.V. solution again, remove the hemostat, and open the primary line clamp. Readjust the flow rate. Document what you've done.

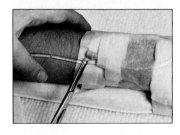

Blood transfusions

How to use a component syringe set

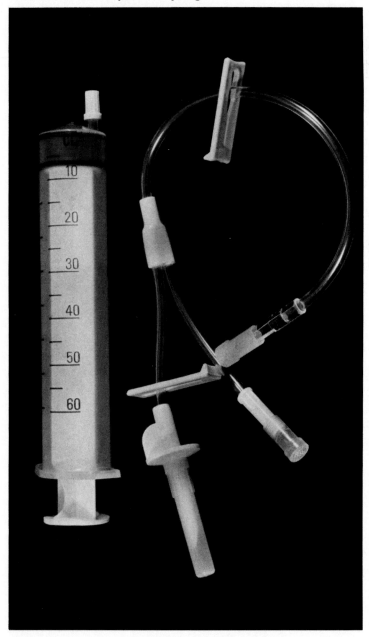

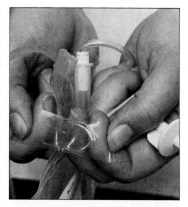

2 Now, pull back the tabs on top of the blood component bag to expose the bag's port.

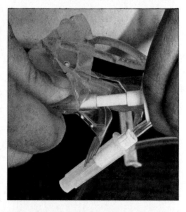

3 Remove the loosened spike cover, and insert the spike in the blood component bag, using a twisting motion.

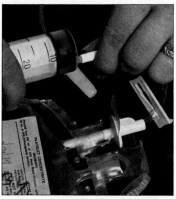

4 Next, remove the cover on the other short length of tubing leading into the Y-connector. Attach a syringe to the end of this tubing, as shown in this photo.

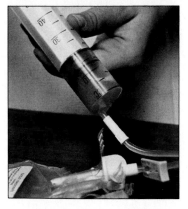

5 Open the clamp above the Y-connector and draw up to 50 ml platelets or cryoprecipitates into the syringe. Close this clamp.

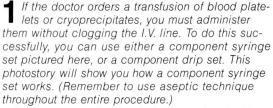

1 *If the doctor orders a transfusion of blood platelets or cryoprecipitates, you must administer them without clogging the I.V. line. To do this successfully, you can use either a component syringe set pictured here, or a component drip set. This photostory will show you how a component syringe set works. (Remember to use aseptic technique throughout the entire procedure.)*

As you can see in this photo, the syringe set has two slide clamps: one just below the bag spike, and the other just below the Y-connector. Close both clamps before you begin the procedure. Then, loosen the cover on the bag spike to prepare it for connection with the blood component bag.

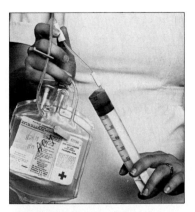

6 Now, open the clamp just *below* the Y-connector. Hold the syringe upright, and prime the tubing. After you've expelled all trapped air, close this clamp.

Now, you're ready to connect the line to the patient. Turn to page 117 to find which method to use for your patient.

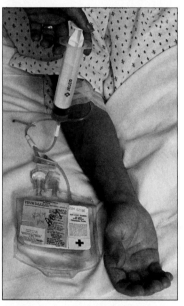

7 After the line's connected, open the clamp below the Y-connector, and begin infusing the blood component at the desired rate. *Important:* If you're administering platelets, deliver the component as fast as possible to prevent clumping.

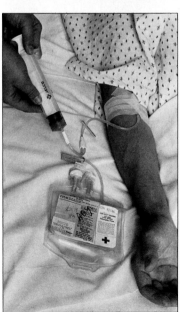

8 When you've delivered all the blood component in the syringe, close the clamp below the Y-connector, and open the clamp above it. Then, pull back on the syringe plunger. This way, you'll draw what remains in the bag into the syringe. When the bag is completely empty, close the clamp above the Y-connector, and open the clamp below it. Infuse the remaining blood component into your patient.

Note: What if you're delivering more than one unit? Disconnect the empty component bag, and flush the line with normal saline solution to test the patency of the vein. Then, spike another blood component bag, and repeat the procedure, starting at step 5.

How to use a component drip set

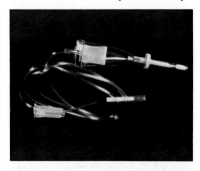

1 *We've shown you how a component syringe set works. Now you'll find out how to use a component drip set.* Here's what the set looks like. Before you begin, make sure the flow rate clamp's positioned just below the drip chamber. Close it. Then, loosen the spike cover.

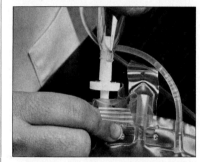

2 Expose the port on the blood component bag. To do this, grasp the tabs at the top of the bag, and pull them back. Remove the spike cover. Insert the spike into the port, using a twisting motion. Make sure it's securely in place.

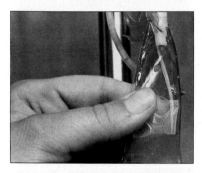

3 Now, remove the needle adapter cover. As you hold the bag upright, open the clamp. Squeeze the combination drip chamber/filter until it's partially filled with the blood component. Then, close the clamp again, and hang the set.

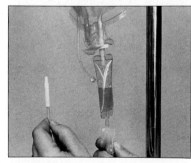

4 If the patient already has an I.V. line in place, attach an 18G needle to the end of the tubing. Holding the needle upright, open the clamp once again to prime the tubing and to expel any trapped air. Then, close the clamp.

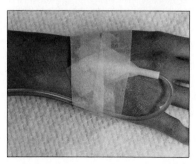

5 Insert the needle into the secondary port. However, be sure to flush the line with normal saline solution first (see page 117).

If the patient doesn't have an I.V. line in place, perform venipuncture, as described on page 31. This photo shows how the site should look after your final taping.

Blood transfusions

Transfusion risks: Immediate reactions

As you probably know, immediate reactions can occur during, immediately after, or up to 96 hours after any blood transfusion. They're primarily caused by incompatibility, contaminated blood, or too rapid an infusion.

Study this chart. You'll learn what to look for, how to treat the reactions, and how to prevent them from happening again.

Reaction	Cause	Signs and symptoms	Treatment	Prevention
Hemolytic (uncommon but possibly fatal)	ABO or Rh incompatibility, or improper storage	Chills, fever, low back pain, chest pain, hypotension, nausea, vomiting, and bleeding abnormalities	Keep the vein open by connecting a secondary line of normal saline solution to the blood line. Correct shock by administering oxygen, fluids, and epinephrine as ordered by the doctor. Maintain renal circulation by administering mannitol (Osmitrol*) or furosemide (Lasix*, Novosemide**). Collect blood and urine samples for lab. Blood will show hemolysis, and urine will contain hemoglobin. Carefully record intake and output after discontinuation of blood. Watch for diuresis and/or oliguria.	Minimize the risk of hemolytic reaction by: • double-checking the patient's identification and blood type to make sure blood is compatible • beginning transfusion slowly • remaining with patient for the first 20 minutes of the transfusion.
Febrile (common but not serious)	Presence of bacterial lipopolysaccharides	From mild chills, fever, to extreme symptoms resembling hemolytic reaction.	For mild cases, administer antipyretics and antihistamines as ordered. For severe cases, treat like hemolytic reaction	Minimize the risk of febrile reaction by: • keeping patient covered and warm • using saline-washed red blood cells or frozen saline-washed packed cells • administering antipyretic medications with the blood. *Important:* Never add antihistamines to the blood bag.
Allergic (common but not serious)	Atopic substance in blood	Pruritus and urticaria, occasional facial swelling, chills, fever, nausea, vomiting	Notify doctor. Administer parenteral antihistamines or, for more serious cases, epinephrine or steroids, as ordered.	Minimize the risk of allergic reaction by: • determining if the patient reacted allergically to previous transfusions. If he did, he has a two-in-three chance of experiencing it again.
Plasma protein incompatibility (uncommon but serious)	IgA incompatibility	Flushing, abdominal pain, diarrhea, chills, fever, dyspnea, hypotension	Treat for shock by administering oxygen, fluids, and epinephrine, as ordered. Sometimes steroids are administered.	Minimize the risk of plasma protein incompatibility reaction by: • transfusing only IgA-deficient blood or well-washed red cells.
Blood contamination (uncommon but serious)	Presence of gram-negative *Pseudomonas*, coliform or achromobacteria	Chills, fever, vomiting, diarrhea, shock	Treat with antibiotics and steroids, as ordered.	Minimize the risk of blood contamination by: • using air-free, touch-free methods to draw and deliver blood • maintaining strict storage control • using aseptic technique when warming infusion • changing the filter and tubing every 4 hours, and the blood at least every 4 hours.
Circulatory overload (common and treatable)	Too large an infusion	Engorged neck veins; constricted chest, with breathing difficulties; flushed feeling; moist rales; eventually acute edema	Keep the primary line open with 5% dextrose in water (not saline solution). Notify doctor immediately for possible administration of diuretics, rotating tourniquets, or phlebotomy therapy.	Minimize the risk of overload by: • using packed red cells instead of whole blood • infusing at a reduced rate for high-risk patient • keeping the patient warm and in a sitting position • using a diuretic when you begin the transfusion.
Air embolism (uncommon but possibly fatal)	Air in bloodstream via tubing	Blood foaming in heart, with subsequent pumping inability, causing shock	Treat for shock. Turn patient on his left side, with his head down.	Minimize the risk of air embolism by: • expelling air from tubing before starting transfusion • not allowing the blood bag to run dry.

*Available in the United States and in Canada.
**Available only in Canada.

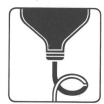

Troubleshooting transfusion problems

You can give your patient the best care possible during a transfusion and still encounter problems. But if you anticipate some of the more common difficulties and know how to deal with them, you can manage the situation well. For example, do you know what to do:

If the transfusion stops running?
• Check the distance between the I.V. container and the insertion site. Make sure it's at least 3' (1 m) above the site.
• Check the flow clamp to make sure it's open.
• Observe the filter to see if it's completely immersed in blood.
• Rock the bag back and forth gently to agitate blood cells that may have settled to the bottom.
• Squeeze the tubing and flashbulb to get the fluid moving again.
• Untape the dressing over the insertion site, and make sure the needle or catheter's still correctly placed in the vein. Reposition it, if necessary.
• If you're using a Y-set, open the saline solution line to dilute the blood and facilitate its flow.

If a hematoma's developing at the needle site?
• Stop the infusion immediately.
• Remove the needle or catheter, and cap the tubing with a new needle and guard.
• Notify the doctor. He'll probably want you to place ice on the site for 24 hours; after that, warm compresses.
• Promote reabsorption of the hematoma by gently exercising the involved limb.
• Document what you've done and observed.

If the blood bag's empty and the new unit hasn't arrived from the blood bank?
• Hang a container of normal saline solution (if you haven't already), and administer it slowly until the new unit arrives.
• If you're using a Y-set, close the blood line clamp, open the saline solution line clamp, and let the saline solution run slowly until the new unit arrives. Make sure you decrease the flow rate or clamp the line before you attach the new unit of blood.

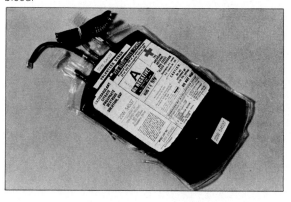

Caring for your patient
Before you transfuse blood, get to know your hospital's policies and procedures concerning transfusions. Then, follow these guidelines to protect your patient:

Always stay with your patient during the first 15 minutes of any blood transfusion. Observe his reaction carefully. Know what to do if complications arise. For example, suppose he starts to shiver and complains that he's cold. For a patient receiving large amounts of blood, this is a common sensation, although it could signal a transfusion reaction. Carefully assess the cause. If it's not a transfusion reaction, counteract the patient's chilled sensations by providing him with blankets. Or, increase the room temperature.

Keeping your patient warm will also increase his peripheral circulation and warm his extremities.

You can avoid many problems connected with blood transfusions by involving the patient in his own care. Instruct him, for instance, on how he can help protect the insertion site. (For details on this, see page 60.)

Remember, too, that the patient and his family will probably be anxious and frightened. Many people associate blood transfusions with serious illness. Do what you can to ease their stress. Encourage questions and answer them honestly. Correct misconceptions, but don't mislead your patient or his family by minimizing the importance of the therapy. Explain the procedure in simple terms so they understand what's happening.

Show that you care in other ways, too. For example, if blood accidentally stains the bed linen, get fresh linen *as soon as possible.* Cover the stain with a towel or pad only as a temporary measure.

Encouraging voluntary blood donations
If your patient needs a blood transfusion, he can expect it to be expensive. But you can suggest a way his family and friends can help him cut that cost. Encourage them to become volunteer blood donors. Then, the blood your patient receives will be free, even though the administration fees will remain the same.

Start your explanation of the volunteer blood donor program by asking if they're already enrolled in a program at either their company or a religious institution. If they're not, suggest they contact a Red Cross center. Explain how a trained staff member draws each donor's blood with a gravity collection set. (If you're not sure how this method works, read the details on page 137.) Remind them that it's simple, almost painless, and relatively hazard-free.

As you may know, almost anyone between ages 18 and 59 can donate blood. But, a person's ineligible if he's receiving medication, has an infectious disease, or has traveled in a malarial area within the past 3 years. A healthy, eligible adult can donate a pint of blood once every 2 months. However, only about 3% of the eligible donors in the United States give blood annually.

Because of this, blood banks frequently replenish their supplies with purchased blood. And when they do, they risk collecting blood that's unhealthy. With purchased blood the chances of transmitting disease are up to ten times greater than with donated blood.

Encourage eligible donors to give blood whenever possible. Make sure you know the location of local blood collection centers, and keep printed information about them handy.

Blood transfusions

Managing a built-in blood pump

1 *If your patient needs large amounts of blood fast, use a blood pump. You have two types of pumps to choose from: a pump that's built into the line, like the one shown here, or a pump that you slip onto the blood bag. The following photos will show you how to use the built-in pump, which operates with manual pressure. (You'll find out how to use the other type of blood pump on page 128.)*
Begin by closing the upper and lower flow clamps. Remove the spike cover.

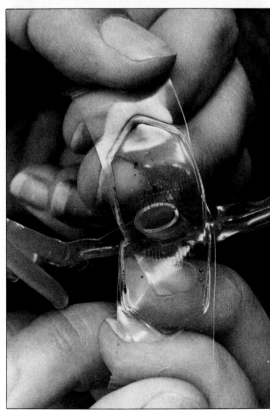

2 Holding the blood bag securely, pull back the two tabs at the top to expose the port. Insert the spike with a twisting motion, making sure it's snug. *Important:* Don't touch the port or you'll contaminate it.

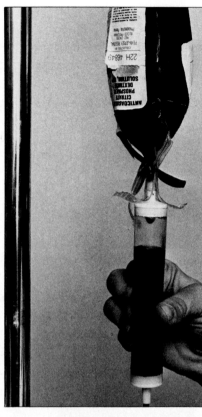

3 Squeeze the combination drip chamber/filter until it begins to fill. Continue squeezing it until the filter's completely immersed in blood. Tap the chamber to expel any trapped air bubbles.

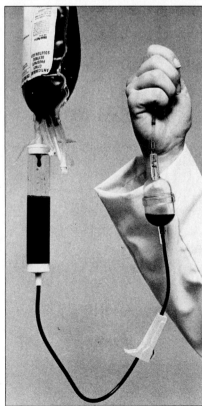

4 Invert the lower pump chamber, as the nurse is doing in this photo. Open both clamps.

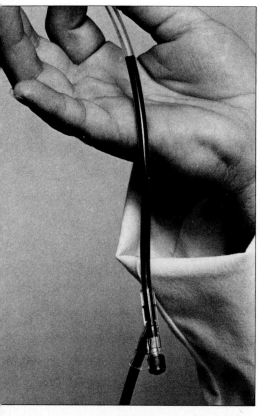

5 Holding the needle adapter upright, prime the tubing. Make sure you expel any trapped air bubbles.

Now, close the lower clamp. If the patient does not have a primary I.V. line in place at that time, perform a venipuncture, following the procedure on page 31.

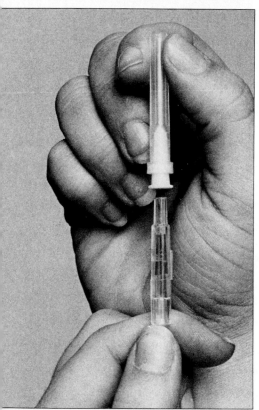

6 However, if the patient already has a primary I.V. line, attach a needle to the blood pump line, as this photo shows. Then, connect the blood pump line to the primary I.V. line, using the same method outlined on page 117.

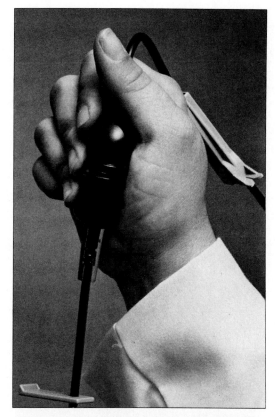

7 Now, you're ready to administer the blood, using this pump. Open both clamps all the way. Apply manual pressure by squeezing and releasing the pump chamber. This forces blood down the tubing.

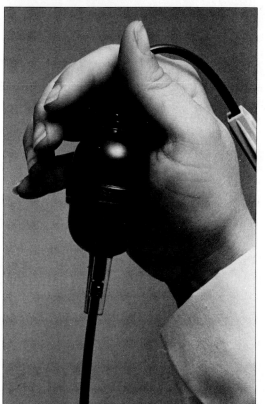

8 Be sure to let the pump chamber refill completely before squeezing and releasing it again. Continue doing this until the blood bag is empty.

Note: If you want to discontinue using the pump to administer the blood before the blood bag is completely emptied, simply stop pumping and adjust the flow rate as you would for normal straight-line administration.

Blood transfusions

More about blood pumps: The slip-on type

1 *Pictured below is another type of pump you can use when you want to administer large amounts of blood quickly. As you'll soon see, it slips right over the blood bag. To use it correctly, follow these instructions:* First, insert the spike of the blood administration set into the blood bag and prime the tubing as you would for a straight-line blood set.

2 Now, insert your hand into the pump envelope, and pull the blood bag up through the center opening, as shown here.

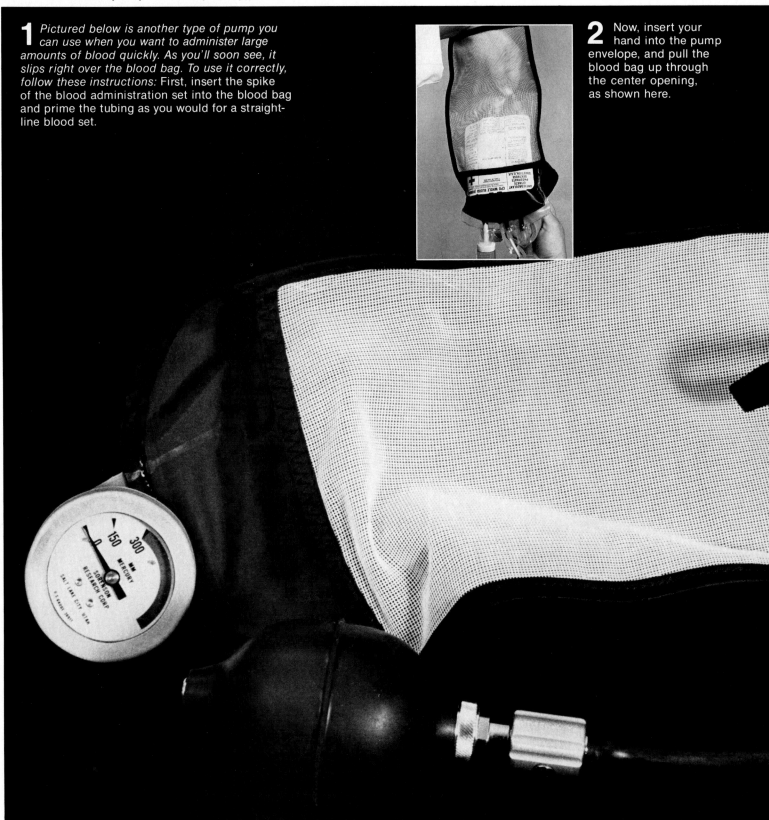

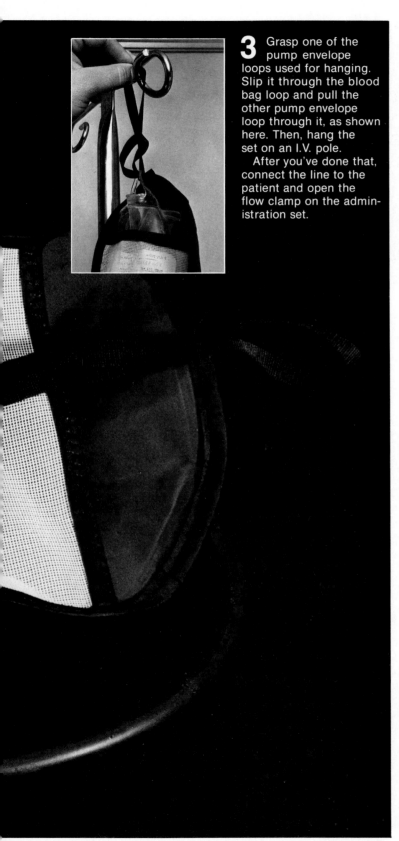

3 Grasp one of the pump envelope loops used for hanging. Slip it through the blood bag loop and pull the other pump envelope loop through it, as shown here. Then, hang the set on an I.V. pole.

After you've done that, connect the line to the patient and open the flow clamp on the administration set.

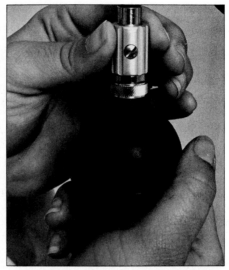

4 Open the screw clamp on the pump by turning it counterclockwise.

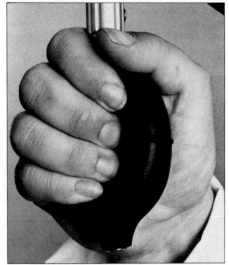

5 Squeeze the bulb of the pump until you've reached the desired flow rate. *Caution:* Don't let the pressure gauge needle on the pump go into the red area. At that level, the pressure's so great it may damage the red blood cells or cause the line to disconnect.

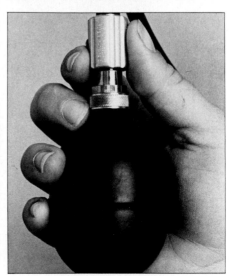

6 Now, turn the screw clamp clockwise to maintain a constant pressure rate. Repeat the procedure outlined above with each new blood bag. Remember, as the bag empties, pressure decreases. Check the flow rate and readjust the flow clamp, as necessary. Observe the venipuncture site carefully. If the vein's too small to accept blood under pressure, the blood may infiltrate the skin.

Blood transfusions

Using a blood-warming coil

1 *Suppose you're caring for a patient who suddenly needs a massive blood transfusion; for example, one who develops extensive gastrointestinal bleeding, or ruptures an abdominal aortic aneurysm. Be sure to warm the blood before you administer it. If you infuse cold blood, the patient may go into shock. To warm a large amount of blood, you can use a blood-warming coil, like the one in this photo, or you can use an electric blood warmer. In this photostory, we'll show you how to use a blood-warming coil.*

Begin by following the procedure outlined for straight-line blood sets, on page 116. Stop when you reach the instructions for hanging the set.

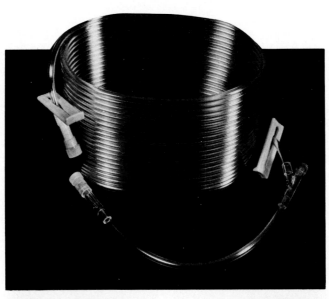

2 Then, using aseptic technique, remove the blood-warming coil from its sterile wrapper, and close the clamps. Make sure the clamp on the straight-line blood set is closed too. When you've completed this, attach the blood line's male adapter to the coil's female adapter. Then, attach the needle to the other end of the coil.

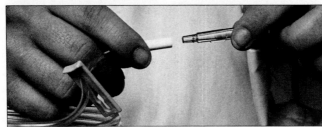

3 Open the straight-line blood clamp and the two coil clamps to prime the tubing. Allow plenty of time for the coil to fill. Then, close the slide clamp nearest the needle.

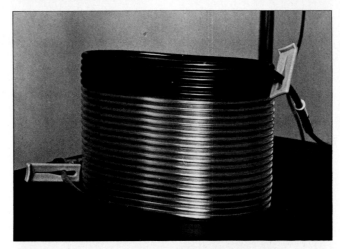

4 To make the coil work properly, you'll have to immerse it in a basin of water warmed to 99° F. (37.6° C.). Make sure the adapters stay dry during this part of the procedure. Otherwise, water may get into the tubing and contaminate the entire setup.

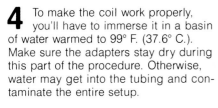

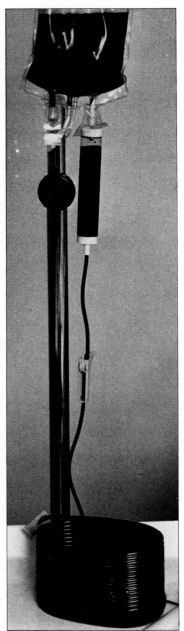

5 Next, perform venipuncture on the patient, or insert the needle into the secondary port of the primary line. Flush the primary line with normal saline solution. Open the blood line's slide clamp, and adjust the flow rate. When the blood bag empties, flush the coil with normal saline solution so you don't waste any blood in the line.

Replace the coil after 24 hours. Discard the old one.

Using an electric blood warmer

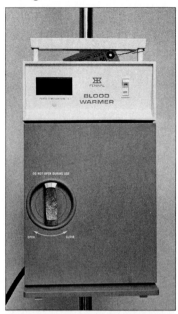

1 *You've already found out how to use a blood-warming coil when you're giving a massive blood transfusion. Now, we'll show you how to use an electric blood warmer, which also must be done using aseptic technique.*

First, attach the blood warmer to an I.V. pole or place it on a bedside table so that it's at mattress height. Plug it into an electrical outlet, but don't turn it on. Instead, prepare and hang a Y-set with a blood bag and normal saline solution. (For details on how to do this, see page 120.) Keep the blood line clamp on the Y-set closed. Remove the cover from the Y-set's needle adapter. Prime the tubing with saline solution, and then replace the cover.

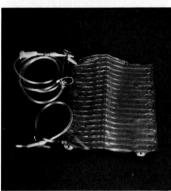

2 Now, you're ready to put the blood-warming bag inside the blood warmer. As you can see in this photo, the warming bag has two leads: one at the bottom, which connects to the primed Y-set; and one at the top, which connects to the patient. Note that the top lead—also called the patient lead—has a special outlet chamber attached to it. Match these leads to the corresponding openings in the electric blood warmer.

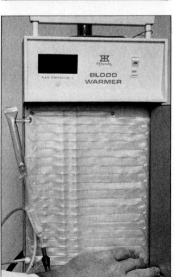

3 Then, insert the warming bag into the warmer, as shown here, and mount it on the support pins. Make sure the bag's flat against the back panel. Secure the top right pin first, then the top left pin, and finally the bottom pins.

Close the blood warmer's door, and secure the latch. Now, turn the warmer on. Give it at least 2 minutes to heat to 99° F. (37° C.), the proper temperature for warming blood.

Important: Once you've secured the door, don't open it again until you've finished the transfusion. If you do, you'll break the vacuum that's been created, and you'll have to begin again with a new warming bag.

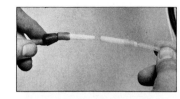

4 While the blood warmer's heating up, connect the Y-set needle adapter to the female adapter on the bottom lead.

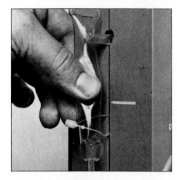

5 When the temperature indicator on the warmer reads 37° C., open the saline-line clamp and the main flow rate clamp to let saline solution fill the blood-warming bag. Squeeze the outlet chamber on the patient lead until it's flat, and then hold it, as shown in this photo.

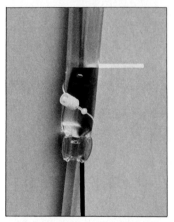

6 The moment saline solution appears in the patient lead chamber, close the main flow rate clamp and release your hold on the chamber. The vacuum you've created in the chamber will automatically cause it to fill halfway with saline solution. Then, remove the adapter cover on the end of the patient lead. Open the clamp on the patient lead, and expel any air that remains in the line. Close the clamp again, and recap the line.

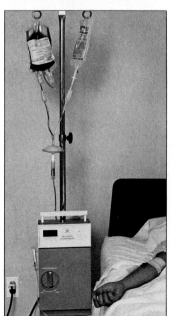

7 Perform venipuncture, following the procedure outlined on page 31. Now, close the saline solution line clamp on the Y-set, and open both the blood line clamp and the main flow rate clamp to start the blood transfusion. Use the main flow rate clamp to adjust and regulate the infusion rate. After the blood's completely infused, open the saline solution line clamp, and flush the warming bag and the tubing. This will clear out any remaining blood.

Important: Take care not to puncture the tubing or the outlet chamber on the patient lead at any time during the transfusion or you may cause an air embolism. And always discard the warming bag after one use.

Blood transfusions

COMPLICATIONS

Transfusion risks: When administering massive amounts

Infusing large amounts of blood naturally carries greater risks than infusing single units. But did you know the complications don't result as much from the large volume as from the necessity for using stored blood? Do what you can to protect your patient against these possible complications. Study this chart, and take the suggested precautions.

Reaction	Cause	Signs and symptoms	Treatment	Prevention
Bleeding tendencies	Low platelet count in stored blood, causing dilutional thrombocytopenia	Abnormal bleeding, and oozing from raw or cut surfaces	Administer platelets, as ordered by doctor.	Use only fresh blood (less than 7 days old, if possible).
Hypocalcemia	A reaction to toxic proportions of citrate, which is used as a preservative in blood. Either the citrate ion combines with calcium, causing a calcium deficiency, or normal citrate metabolism is hindered by hepatic disease.	Tingling sensation in fingers, muscle cramps, convulsions, hypotension, shock, tetany, or cardiac arrest	Slowly administer calcium chloride I.V., as ordered by doctor.	Monitor calcium levels carefully, especially if patient has hepatic disease. Follow the doctor's orders for treatment. Use only frozen saline-washed cells. As you know, the plasma has been removed from these cells, which lowers the citrate content.
Increased oxygen affinity	A decreased level of 2,3,DPG in stored blood, causing an increase in the oxygen's hemoglobin affinity. When that happens, oxygen stays in the patient's bloodstream and isn't released into his tissues.	Depressed respirations, especially in patients with chronic lung disease, who depend on their low oxygen level to breathe.	Monitor arterial blood gas measurements, and give respiratory support, as needed.	Use only red blood cells or fresh blood, if possible.
Potassium intoxication	An abnormally high potassium level in stored plasma, caused by red blood cell lysis	Renal failure; nausea; diarrhea; vague muscle weakness; slow or irregular heart beat; paresthesis of hands, face, tongue. EKG changes: tall, peaked T waves	Administer hypertonic Kayexalate orally or by enema, as ordered.	Use only red blood cells, fresh frozen plasma, or blood stored for less than 7 days, especially if patient has renal failure.
Elevated blood ammonia level	An increased level of ammonia in stored blood	Forgetfulness, confusion	Decrease amount of protein in diet. If the doctor orders, give neomycin sulfate (Mycifradin Sulfate*, Neobiotic) when necessary.	Use only red blood cells, fresh frozen plasma, or blood stored less than 7 days, especially if patient has hepatic disease.
Hemosiderosis	Increased hemosiderin (iron-containing pigment) from red blood cell destruction	Iron plasma level greater than 200 mg per l00 ml	Perform a phlebotomy to remove excess iron.	Don't administer blood unless it's absolutely necessary.
Hypothermia	Large volume of blood administered at too cold a temperature	Decreased temperature, chills, and possible cardiac arrest	Call the doctor. Warm the patient with blankets.	Minimize the risk of hypothermia by warming blood before giving massive transfusion.

*Available in the United States and in Canada.

COMPLICATIONS

Transfusion risks: Transmittable diseases

You can never be sure the blood you're infusing is disease-free. While blood donated by volunteers usually poses fewer risks than blood that's been purchased from the donor, you must be careful in either case. This chart will help you identify some of the diseases that can be transmitted by transfusion, tell you how to treat them effectively, and how to prevent them from occurring in other patients.

Disease	Cause	Incubation time	How to confirm	How to treat	How to prevent
Hepatitis	Presence of hepatitis B in blood (greatest risk in pooled plasma, fibrinogen, concentrates of Factors VIII and IX; no risk in immune serum, globulin, PPF, normal serum albumin)	2 weeks to 6 months	Make sure the blood is tested for hepatitis B antigens before administering it. Patient will have anorexia, vomiting, abdominal discomfort, enlarged liver, diarrhea, headache, fever, and jaundice.	Isolation, gamma globulin therapy, supportive treatment.	Select reliable, healthy blood donors. Conduct epidemologic follow-ups of suspected cases to potential carriers. Conduct radioimmunoassays for hepatitis B on all donor blood products. Make sure blood is tested for the Australia antigen.
Malaria	Presence of protozoan parasites within the red blood cells	2 weeks to 4 months	Test blood for plasmodium species.	Administer quinine sulfate (Coco-Quinine) or chloroquine phosphate (Aralen Phosphate*).	Select only those donors who have not lived in endemic areas or have not taken antimalarial drugs for at least 3 years.
Syphilis	Spirochetemia caused by *Treponema pallidum*	4 to 18 weeks	Check blood for syphilis with a serologic test, but don't consider results absolutely reliable. You can, however, consider a chancre positive proof of syphilis.	Administer penicillin therapy.	Don't administer blood unless it's been tested and refrigerated for at least 2 days at 39.2° F. (4° C.) to kill spirochetes.
Viral syndrome	Presence of cytomegalovirus (CMV) or Epstein-Barr virus in blood	2 to 5 weeks	The patient will show signs of fever; hepatitis to varying degrees, with or without jaundice; atypical lymphocytosis; rash.	No specific therapy; let the reactions run their course.	Select only those donors who are free from recent viral symptoms.

*Available in the United States and in Canada.

Blood transfusions

Documenting a blood transfusion correctly

The procedure for documenting a blood transfusion begins even before any blood is administered. Don't open the blood line until you've recorded the patient's base-line vital signs on his chart. Then, when you've transfused the blood for at least 10 minutes, check his vital signs again. You'll notice changes if the patient's developing complications from the transfusion (for example, hemolysis).

Recheck the patient's vital signs after 1 hour; then again when the transfusion's completed. Document this information, along with your other observations about the procedure. Include the number and contents of the unit, the time it was hung, its flow rate, and absorption site. Examine the sample chart to the right.

Make sure you also complete the requisition form attached to the blood unit by filling in the time the transfusion was completed and the amount transfused. Attach one copy of the form to the patient's chart, along with the lab's blood type report. Return the other copy to the blood bank, with the empty blood bag. If your hospital also keeps a master blood transfusion record, document all relevant information on that also.

Date	Time	No.	Problem	
6-25-80	9 AM	3	Blood loss from GI tract	S – Patient complains of nausea.
				O – No further vomiting of blood as previously reported. Hgb. 8.8 VS 97-100-24 B/P 104/60
				A – No overt bleeding.
				P – T&C order 2 units of packed RBCs sent to lab.
	9:45 AM			S – Patient says nausea has lessened
				O – Patient pale; skin warm and dry; conjunctiva pale. VS 97-84-16 B/P 112/70 #1 unit Packed RBCs #4538 started in ® antecubital space with an 18G Jelco. Absorbing at 32# gtts per minute via the IVAC pump.
				A – Transfusion started without difficulty; no problem at I.V. site.
				P – Reassess patient's condition in 15 minutes.
	10 AM			S – Patient says, "I feel better now that I'm getting this blood."
				O – VS 97²-88-18 B/P 116/70 Blood absorbing without difficulty. Site O.K.
				A – No signs of transfusion reaction at this time.
				P – Recheck VS, including temperature, in 1 hour. M. Klevence RN.

Phlebotomy

Suppose you're giving your patient a massive transfusion and he develops a circulatory overload. You may have to perform a phlebotomy. Do you know how? You can use either of two methods: the vacuum collection set or the gravity collection set. Learn about them by reading the next few pages.

INDICATIONS/CONTRAINDICATIONS

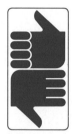

When to perform a phlebotomy

You may be called on to perform a phlebotomy in these cases: to reduce blood volume in a patient with polycythemia or circulatory overload, or to collect blood from a donor. In any of these cases, the basic procedures are the same.

Consider the possibility that your patient has polycythemia if he has an elevated hematocrit (usually 50% or more), or a red blood cell count above 6 million per/cu mm. In such a case, the doctor may want you to perform a phlebotomy to reduce the patient's hematocrit level and maintain it at about 45%. To accomplish this, you'll probably have to repeat the procedure three to six times, drawing 500 ml of blood each time.

Important: Is the polycythemic patient elderly? Or does he have severe arteriosclerosis or heart disease? In such cases, never draw more than 250 ml of blood.

Whenever a phlebotomy's ordered, keep these points in mind:
• Record the patient's vital signs before and after the phlebotomy.
• Stay with the patient throughout the entire procedure. Observe him closely for signs of hypotension; for example, faintness or light-headedness.
• Never perform a phlebotomy if blood loss will jeopardize your patient's health.

The doctor may also choose to do a phlebotomy if the patient has a circulatory overload. As you know, this condition may be caused by too large an infusion of blood. To determine if your patient has a circulatory overload, watch for these danger signs: engorged neck veins, labored breathing, increased blood pressure, and increased pulse rate. Call the doctor immediately. If left untreated, circulatory overload can cause cardiac arrest. The doctor will specify the amount of blood to withdraw during the phlebotomy.

How to use a vacuum collection set

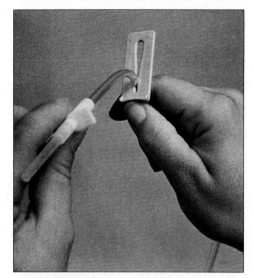

1 *When you're using a vacuum collection set to perform a phlebotomy, begin the procedure as follows:*

Position the patient comfortably. If he's having trouble breathing, put him in a semi-Fowler's or high Fowler's position. Then, take his vital signs and record them.

Next, close the slide clamp on the vacuum collection set. Later, when you spike the container, this will prevent a vacuum loss.

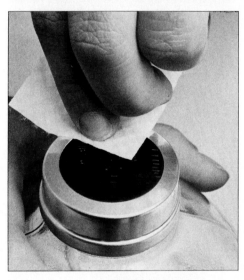

2 Now, prepare the collection bottle for spiking by removing the cap's metal disc. Swab the stopper with alcohol.

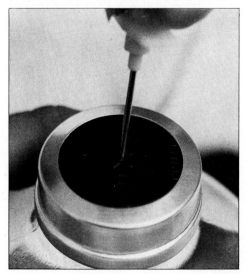

3 Remove the spike guard. Insert the spike through the X on the top of the collection bottle. Then, place the bottle close to the patient. Remove the needle guard. Find a large vein in one of the patient's extremities and perform venipuncture, using the indirect method shown on page 31.

Phlebotomy

How to use a vacuum collection set continued

4 When you get a blood backflow, open the line's slide clamp. Use the clamp to adjust the blood's flow rate. While you're withdrawing the correct amount of blood, observe the patient's color and monitor his vital signs. If you notice any significant changes in his condition (for example, a blood pressure drop), call the doctor.

Nursing tip. Always use a collection bottle that's been flushed with an antifoamant. If you don't, foam may fill the bottle and make it difficult to determine how much blood you've withdrawn.

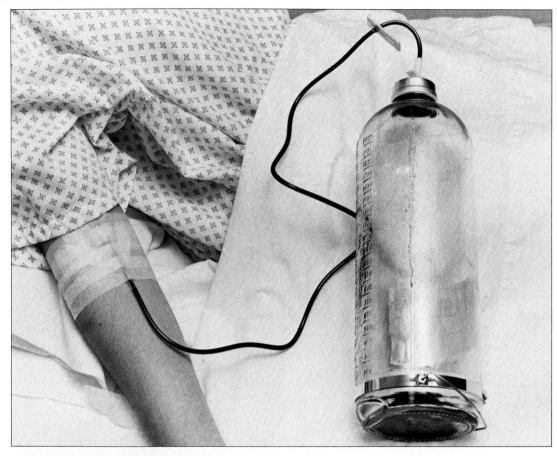

5 When the phlebotomy's completed, close the flow-control clamp. Then, remove the needle from the patient's arm, and apply pressure to the insertion site.

Disconnect the set. Wrap the collection bottle and tubing in a plastic or paper bag, making sure you've first protected (or removed) the needle and spike. Discard the bag in a wastebasket. Don't leave it in full view for patients or visitors to see. Finally, fully document the phlebotomy, following the procedure we've outlined on the right.

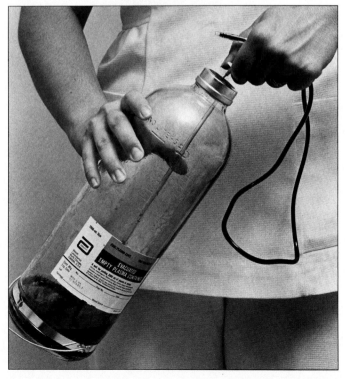

Documenting a phlebotomy

After the phlebotomy, document the following:
• the patient's vital signs and urine output. If there's any significant change, notify the doctor.
• the amount of blood you've removed.
• how well the patient tolerated the procedure.

Later, compare the lab reports on the patient's hemoglobin and hematocrit levels with earlier reports. Document these findings daily for the next few days. Keep the doctor informed.

Note: If the patient's ambulatory, explain that he'll feel light-headed if he changes position suddenly. Tell him, for his own safety, to call you the first time he tries to stand.

How to use a gravity collection set

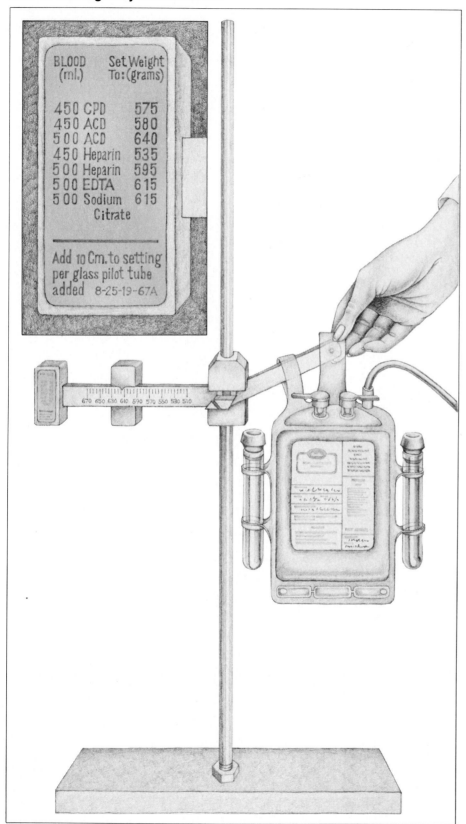

BLOOD   Set.Weight
(ml.)   To:(grams)

450 CPD   575
450 ACD   580
500 ACD   640
450 Heparin   535
500 Heparin   595
500 EDTA   615
500 Sodium   615
    Citrate

Add 10 Cm. to setting
per glass pilot tube
added   8-25-19-67A

On page 135, we explained how to use a vacuum collection set to draw blood. But what if you want to use a gravity collection set instead? Study this photostory to learn how.

First, familiarize yourself with the equipment: a blood bag (complete with tubing and large-bore needle) and a gravity scale to weigh the amount of blood the doctor's ordered withdrawn.

The gravity collection set is generally used to perform a donor phlebotomy, but we'll tell you how to use the set for a therapeutic phlebotomy. Begin by positioning the patient comfortably. Record his vital signs. Then, proceed as follows:

Set the gravity scale for the proper weight, using the guidelines printed on the long arm of the scale (see the inset). To determine the weight, you must know the bag's capacity, as well as the kind of anticoagulant it contains.

What if you want to take a blood sample at the same time you perform the phlebotomy? In this case, attach a pair of glass pilot tubes to the sides of the blood bag, as the nurse has done here. Consult the guidelines on the scale to determine the weight adjustment needed for the added weight of the pilot tubes. Reset the scale accordingly, and hang the bag on the short arm of the scale.

Now, perform the venipuncture, as described in Section 2 of this PHOTOBOOK. Watch for blood backflow. Then, temporarily secure the needle with adhesive tape.

Important: Don't leave the patient unattended at any time during the procedure.

Throughout the procedure, watch the bag closely. When the weight of the blood equals the weight you've set on the scale, the arm holding the bag will fall to a level position. As soon as it does, clamp the tubing close to the needle, using a hemostat. Remove the needle from the patient's arm. To minimize bleeding, apply pressure to the site with a 2" x 2" sterile gauze pad. Then, cover the site with an adhesive bandage strip.

If you want a blood sample, insert the needle into the stopper of one of the pilot tubes, as shown here. When you release the hemostat, the tube will fill with blood. Then, clamp the tubing again and withdraw the needle. Repeat this procedure to fill the second pilot tube.

Finally, take the patient's vital signs and record them. Document the procedure, including the information you'd record after a vacuum collection set procedure.

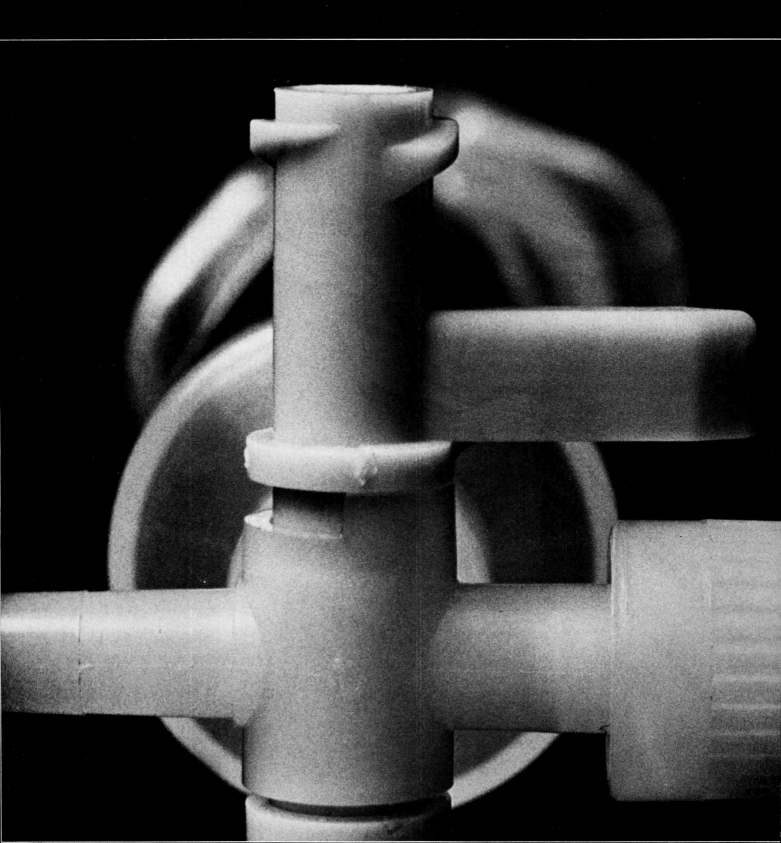

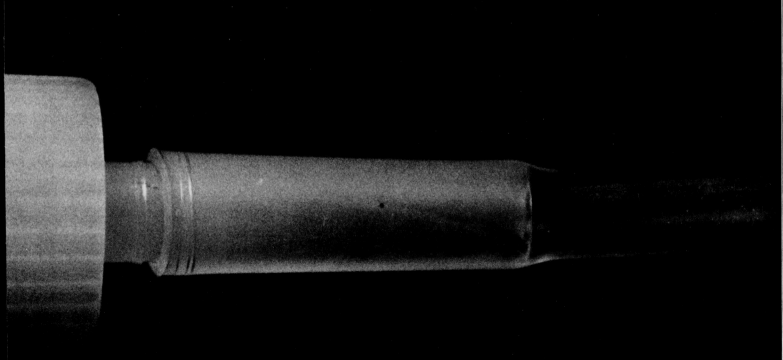

Managing Special Procedures

Central venous pressure
Cutdowns
Umbilical lines

Central venous pressure

As you know, you can use a central line to give hyperalimentation solution or a large dose of an irritating drug. But the line has another important function as well. When threaded into the superior vena cava or the right atrium of the heart, it measures central venous pressure (CVP). CVP readings help you:

- assess the function of the heart's right side
- monitor fluid replacement
- evaluate blood volume.

You've already learned all about central lines (see pages 90 through 97). On the following pages, you'll learn how to take accurate CVP readings.

Helping to insert a central line for measuring CVP

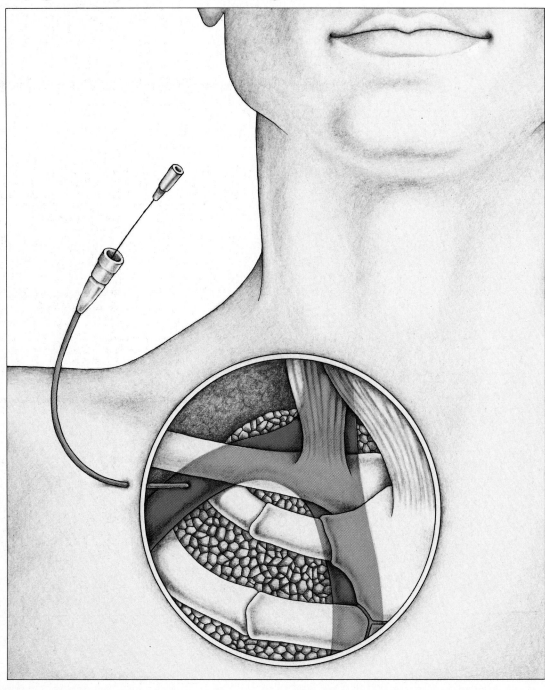

What's the best insertion site for a central line? Most doctors prefer one of the following veins: a subclavian, one in the antecubital fossa, or an internal jugular. The femoral and the saphenous veins are less desirable because they're prone to thrombosis and infection. What's more, CVP readings from these veins may be affected by intra-abdominal pressures.

The procedure for inserting a CVP line is the same as for inserting a central hyperalimentation line. The only difference is that the CVP line is fed further into the vein to the superior vena cava or the right atrium of the heart.

But this variation doesn't change your responsibilities. Turn back to page 94, and review the insertion procedure carefully. Then, when you assist the doctor, keep these particular points in mind:
- Explain the procedure to the patient, and answer his questions. Make sure he's signed a consent form if your hospital requires one.
- Wash your hands thoroughly, and help the doctor maintain sterile technique.
- Position the patient in a 30° Trendelenburg position for a subclavian or jugular insertion. For an insertion in the antecubital fossa, have him lie flat on his back, with his arm outstretched. Position his hand palm up.
- Make sure that the catheter the doctor inserts is radiopaque, and that he confirms correct placement with an X-ray immediately after the procedure.

How to set up a manometer

1 *Suppose your patient's receiving an infusion through a central line. If the doctor orders CVP readings, could you set up a manometer? The following photostory shows you how:*

Begin by washing your hands and assembling your equipment. The manometer we're using in this story has two parts: a reusable metal scale and a disposable length of tubing with a three-way stopcock attached to it. Clamp the scale to the I.V. pole, as shown here.

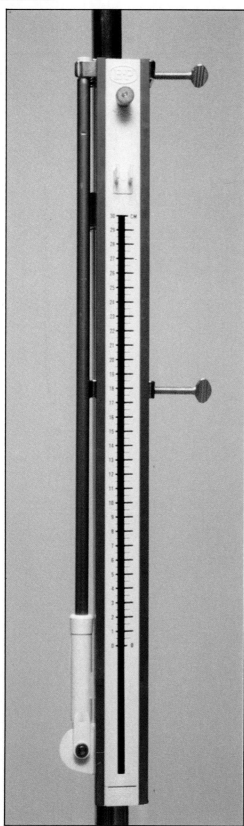

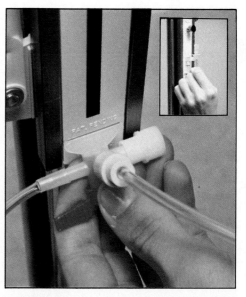

2 To attach the tubing, just snap the stopcock into the bottom of the scale, and stretch the pliable tubing to the top. [Inset] The T-bar attachment at the end of the tubing fits over the hooks at the top of the scale, keeping the tubing taut.

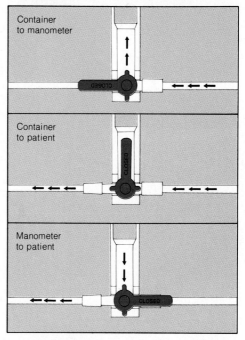

Container to manometer

Container to patient

Manometer to patient

3 Examine this three-way stopcock. By turning it to any of the positions shown here, you can control the direction of fluid flow. Although stopcock designs vary according to manufacturer, this is a common type. Four-way stopcocks are also available. The fourth position blocks off all openings.

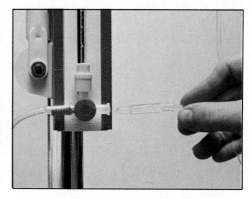

4 When the manometer's in place, turn the stopcock to the CONTAINER-TO-MANOMETER position. Then, connect the I.V. tubing to the open side of the stopcock. Make sure your tubing doesn't feature an in-line filter, because it can distort your reading.

Central venous pressure

How to set up a manometer continued

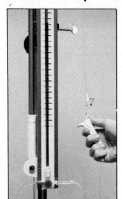

5 Fill the manometer to about the 18 cm mark. Don't fill it to the top, or you'll contaminate the air filter.

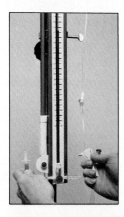

6 Then, turn the stopcock to the CONTAINER-TO-PATIENT position. The solution will then flow from the container through the second piece of tubing, flushing it. Remember, air embolisms are a serious danger with central lines. Take special care to expel all trapped air from the tubing.

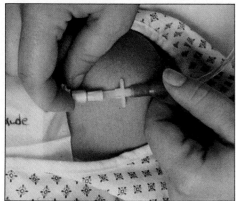

7 Then, close the flow clamp and cap the tubing. Loosen the connector on the I.V. line, and ask the patient to bear down (Valsalva maneuver). Quickly disconnect the old line, uncap the new tubing, and connect it to the catheter.

What if the patient's unconscious and can't do a Valsalva maneuver? Wait until he inhales fully; then quickly connect the tubing. If he's intubated, keep the patient at full inflation while you connect the tubing.

Finally, adjust the flow clamp to slow the I.V. solution infusion rate. Check for blood backflow by lowering the container below the patient's heart.

How to take a CVP reading

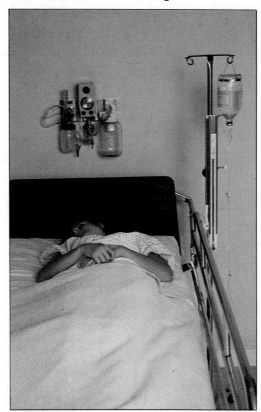

1 *We've shown you how to set up a manometer. Now, after you explain the procedure to the patient, you're ready to take a reading. The following photos show how.*

First, position the patient flat on her back, without a pillow, unless her condition dictates otherwise. (See page 145.) Make sure the I.V. line's open between the patient and container.

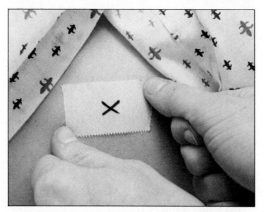

2 As you know, the right atrium is approximately midway between a patient's sternum and her back at the fourth intercostal space, midaxillary. Locate it and mark it with tape and an indelible marker. Remember, all subsequent readings must be taken from the same point.

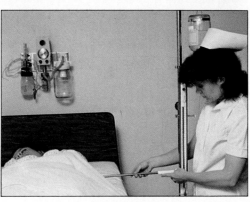

3 Use the arm on the manometer scale to line up the patient's right atrium with the zero point on the scale. *Note:* Some manometer scales are marked with minus numbers below the zero mark. Make sure the arm on the scale is perpendicular to the zero mark, even if you must slide the scale below the metal holder.

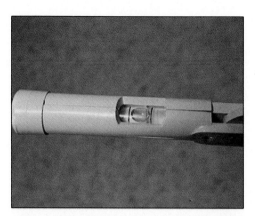

4 How can you be sure the arm is perpendicular to the zero mark? Just center the arm's leveling bubble, as you see here.

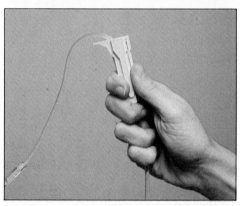

5 Now, check for patency by briefly increasing the flow rate of the I.V. line. If the line's not patent, notify the doctor. *Remember:* Never irrigate a clogged I.V. line. Doing so may force a clot into the patient's bloodstream.

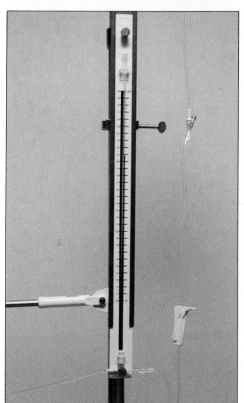

6 Next, turn the stopcock so the I.V. solution runs into the manometer, not the patient. Let the manometer tubing fill slowly, until it's nearly full. However, don't fill it all the way or you'll contaminate the air filter. *Note:* Some manometers have cotton air filters. If this type of filter gets wet, it will produce an inaccurate reading. Replace the manometer and begin again.

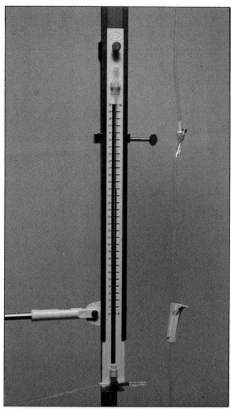

7 Now, turn the stopcock to MANOMETER-TO-PATIENT position. Notice how the fluid drops part of the way down the column. *Nursing tip:* In rare instances, the fluid may not drop because the patient's CVP measurement is higher than the highest reading on the manometer. If this happens, raise the manometer's position on the I.V. pole. Then, adjust your reading accordingly. For example, suppose you raise the manometer 10 cm. Add 10 cm to the reading. Then, document what you've done.

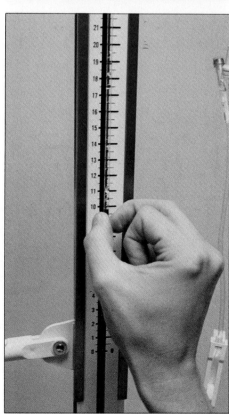

8 When the fluid level comes to rest in the manometer (usually between 5 and 15 cm), tap the manometer column lightly with a finger to eliminate air bubbles that may distort your reading.

Central venous pressure

How to take a CVP reading continued

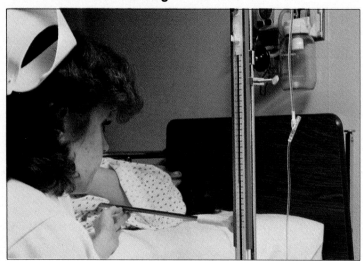

9 Then, look at the meniscus from *eye level.* (If you're not sure what a meniscus is, read the information on the right.) Notice how the fluid rises and falls slightly as the patient breathes.

Nursing tip: If the fluid doesn't fluctuate as the patient breathes, suspect that the end of the catheter is pressed against the vein wall. To remedy this problem, ask the patient to cough. This may be enough to change the catheter's position slightly.

Now, instruct your patient to lie still. Then, note the highest level reached by the fluid and take your reading from the base of the meniscus. *Note:* If your manometer has a small ball floating on the fluid surface, take the reading from the ball's midline.

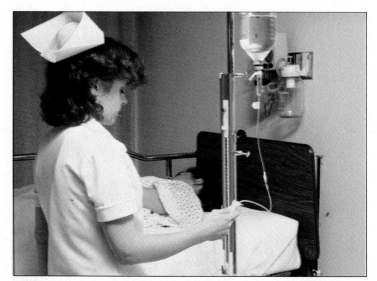

10 To maintain the line's patency, turn the stopcock back to CONTAINER-TO-PATIENT position, and check for blood backflow. Readjust the flow rate. Then, chart and document your reading, including the patient's position, manometer position, time, date, and your name. Secure all connections to minimize the risk of hemorrhage.

Always replace the I.V. container before it empties. If a bottle runs dry, negative pressure generated by central veins may pull air from the empty bottle into the patient's body. And if a bag runs dry, the catheter will clot.

What's a meniscus?

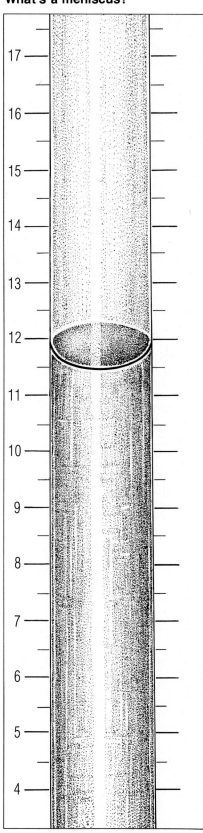

The term meniscus refers to the curved surface of fluid in the manometer's plastic column. When the inside of the column's wet, the fluid climbs up its sides. As a result, the fluid surface is concave. Take your reading from the base of the meniscus, which is represented by the black line in this illustration. (This reading is 11½.) *Important:* To get an accurate reading, look at the base of the meniscus from eye level, even if you must get on your knees.

Using a one-piece manometer

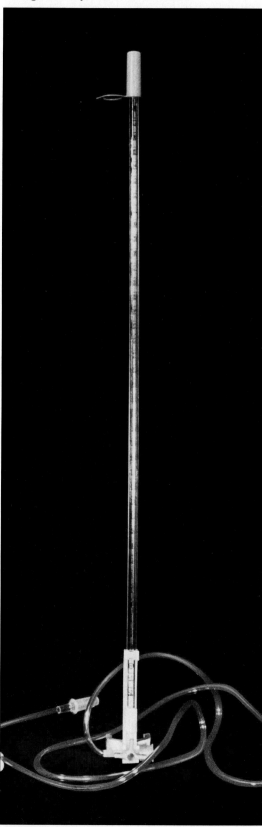

This is a disposable, one-piece manometer. As you can see, the scale is marked on the clear plastic column. Use the plastic C-shaped clip to snap the entire unit on the I.V. pole. If it doesn't snap firmly to the pole, secure it with tape. Remember, if it falls off the pole and the tubing disconnects, the patient will lose blood and run the risk of infection. *Note:* To assure an accurate reading, keep the manometer vertical, even if it's not perfectly flat against the I.V. pole.

How to interpret a CVP reading

Now you know how to take a CVP reading. But do you know how to interpret it and when to take action? Here are some guidelines:

Keep in mind that you can't assess any CVP reading properly until you've established a normal range for your patient. (An average reading is usually between 5 and 15 cm, but this varies from patient to patient.)

To establish a normal range for *your* patient, take a series of measurements at 15-, 30-, and 60-minute intervals. Then, if a reading varies from the range you've established by more than 2 cm, take action. Here's how:

First, check the patient's vital signs. If they seem stable, check the line for patency, and make sure you've followed measurement procedures correctly (see page 142). Remember, a blocked line will cause a false low reading; a loose connection will cause a false high reading.

If you're sure the reading's accurate, notify the doctor. Don't rely on stable vital signs as an indication that all's well. Regular checks of CVP measurements can serve as an early warning system. Why? Because CVP changes may precede observable changes in vital signs. For example, a high reading may signal congestive heart failure, hypervolemia, vasoconstriction, or early stage cardiac tamponade. A low reading, on the other hand, may indicate peripheral blood pooling, hypovolemia, or vasodilation.

If the CVP changes significantly, the doctor will probably order an X-ray to look for changes in the patient's chest condition. He'll also want to determine if the catheter tip has migrated.

COMPLICATIONS

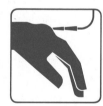

When the patient has special problems

Sometimes you'll have to alter the procedure for a CVP measurement, so you can accommodate your patient's health problems. However, as long as you take all readings under the same conditions, you'll be able to recognize significant changes quickly.

For example, suppose your patient has problems breathing and can't tolerate lying flat. Leave him in a comfortable position, but make sure you put him in the same position for subsequent readings.

Or, perhaps he must be on a ventilator at all times. This will elevate his CVP readings falsely, especially if he's receiving positive end expiratory pressure (PEEP). To allow for this, take *all* readings while the patient's on the ventilator. Then you'll be able to spot significant CVP changes.

Remember to thoroughly document unusual circumstances. This way, the nurse who takes the next reading can maintain consistency.

Cutdowns

Sometimes peripheral veins seem to vanish just when you need them most. Veins may become inaccessible when:
• the patient's in shock and his veins have constricted.
• the patient's had a series of venipunctures and his peripheral veins have collapsed.
• the patient's very thin or elderly and his veins are too small, sclerotic, or fragile.

Under any of these circumstances, the doctor may decide to do a cutdown—a simple surgical technique that exposes the vein so a catheter can be inserted. Once the catheter's in place, it's used for the same purposes as any peripheral I.V. line.

While the doctor performs the cutdown, help him maintain sterile technique. Afterward, care for the patient as you would any patient undergoing I.V. therapy. As always, stay alert for the first signs of I.V. therapy complications, such as infiltration, thrombophlebitis, embolism, or infection. (For details on signs and symptoms, review the chart on pages 58 and 59.)

On these two pages, we'll give you some tips on assisting the doctor and caring for the patient.

Choosing a vein for cutdown

Most veins can be used for a cutdown procedure, even central veins, although this is unusual. The most common choices, however, are the basilic and the cephalic veins of the antecubital fossa. When the cephalic vein is used below the antecubital fossa, the radial bone acts as a natural splint. Femoral and saphenous sites are least desirable, because they're prone to clotting and infection.

Helping the doctor perform a cutdown

1 *When you assist the doctor in performing a cutdown, what should you do first?* As always, wash your hands and double-check the patient's identity. Then, assemble all the equipment the doctor needs: I.V. solution, I.V. tubing, prepping and dressing materials, scalpel, suture materials, a pair of sterile gloves, a cutdown tray, and catheters in assorted sizes. If the doctor plans the cutdown near one of the patient's joints, include a splint and restraints. The doctor will explain the procedure to the patient. See that the patient has signed a consent form.

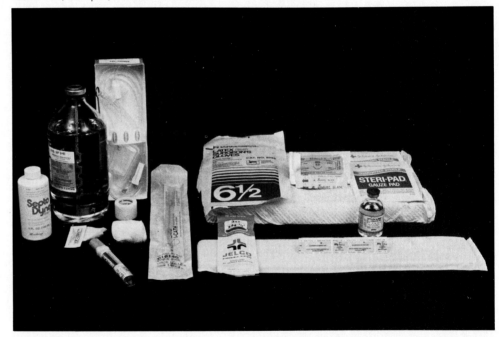

2 Position the patient flat on the bed so the insertion site's fully exposed.
As you see in this photo, the doctor has chosen to do the cutdown on the cephalic vein in the patient's lower arm. Slip a bedsaver pad under the patient to protect the bed. When that's done, the doctor can prep the patient's skin, inject a local anesthetic, and place sterile drapes around the site.

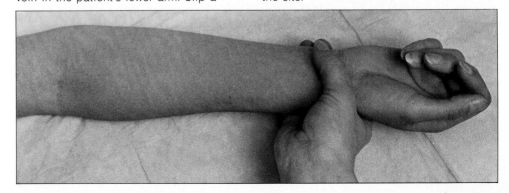

3 Next, he'll make a skin incision to expose the vein. After spreading the incision with a hemostat, he'll stabilize the vein by putting two catgut ties underneath it and pulling them firmly in opposite directions.

After that, he'll make a small incision in the vein's wall, as shown here.

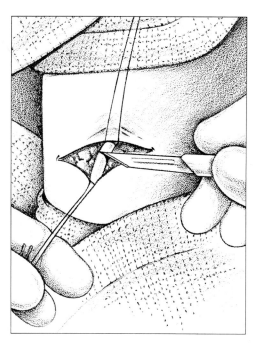

4 Now, the doctor will thread the correct size catheter into the exposed vein, inserting it almost to the hub.

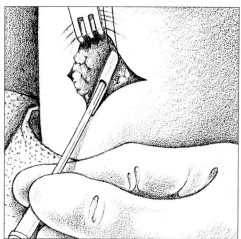

5 Then, attach the catheter to the infusion set and adjust the flow rate. *Note:* If the doctor's used a preshaped drape, fold it back on itself before you attach the catheter to the infusion set. Later, you or the doctor can remove the drape without disconnecting the tubing.

Stand by as the doctor sutures the skin.

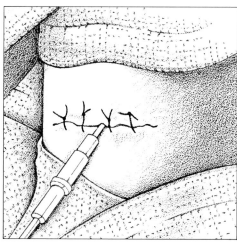

6 Apply antimicrobial ointment to the insertion site. Then, tape the catheter in place to prevent stress on the sutures. If possible, use sterile tape to reduce the risk of contamination. Remove the drape.

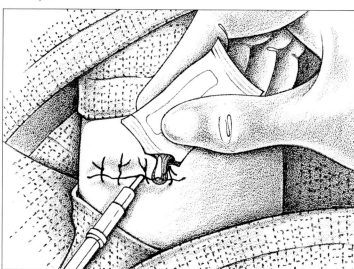

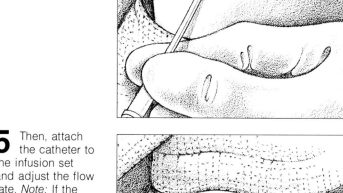

7 Now, apply a 2" x 2" sterile gauze pad over the site and tape securely. Change the dressing daily.

Thoroughly document the procedure in your nurses' notes. Include the date and time, insertion site, catheter size, and doctor's initials. Mark the dressing, tubing, and container, as explained on page 43.

Removing a cutdown catheter

If your hospital permits you to remove a cutdown catheter, you can follow almost the same procedure you'd use to remove a central line (see page 104). However, keep these important differences in mind:

• In the cutdown procedure, remove only the retaining sutures the doctor may have used to secure the catheter. Take care not to nick the catheter or cut any skin sutures.

• After you've removed the catheter, press a 2" x 2" sterile gauze pad to the site to stop the bleeding. Then, apply antimicrobial ointment, and firmly tape another 2" x 2" sterile gauze pad over the site. You won't need a pressure bandage, because the skin sutures will hold the incision closed.

• Ask the doctor when he wants the skin sutures removed. Include that information in your nurses' notes.

Umbilical lines

Someday you may have to care for a seriously ill infant who's receiving medication, fluid, or an exchange blood transfusion through an umbilical catheter. Do you know why an umbilical line is usually preferred to a peripheral one if the patient's an infant? How does the doctor decide whether to choose the vein or one of the arteries in the umbilical cord? What danger signs should you watch for during the procedure? What kind of care will the infant need later? If you're not sure, read the following pages carefully.

Gathering umbilical line equipment

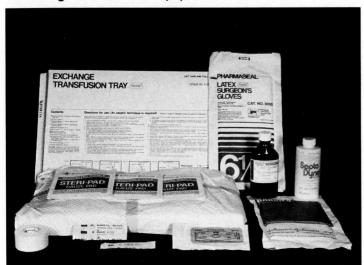

If you're assisting the doctor with an umbilical line insertion, begin by gathering all the equipment shown in this photo. An umbilical line tray contains all the basic instruments he'll need, including an assortment of radiopaque catheters in French sizes 3.5, 5.0, and 8.0. If the infant needs an exchange blood transfusion, make sure you also have a transfusion tray. This tray contains this additional equipment: a special blood administration set, a blood waste bag, and a vial of 10% calcium gluconate. With either tray, you'll need additional sterile gauze pads.

To keep the infant warm during the procedure, make sure you also have a radiant heater or heating blanket.

Now, pick up the blood the doctor's ordered from the lab. As you probably know, this blood must be crossmatched with both the infant's and mother's blood. (For more details on your responsibilities during blood administration, see page 113.) Remember, if he'll be inserting the catheter into an umbilical artery, he'll also need an I.V. infusion pump and an administration set. To find out how to set up a pump, see page 51.

Here's another important preliminary precaution: Make sure you have an oxygen source and emergency equipment nearby.

Artery or vein: How the doctor chooses

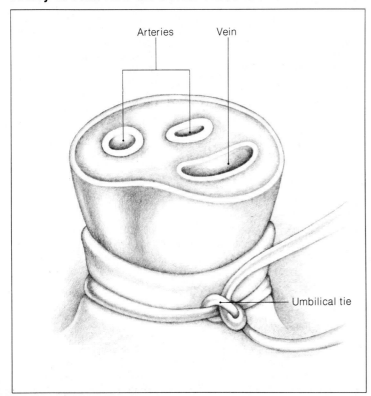

Arteries   Vein

Umbilical tie

In a newborn infant, I.V. therapy may be given through the vein or the arteries of the umbilical cord. Since the single vein in the cord is larger than either of the two arteries, insertion in the vein is usually easier, with less risk of vascular spasm. However, a venous line is only used for these limited purposes:
• To give lifesaving drugs and I.V. solutions in the delivery room when there's no time to establish a peripheral I.V. line or an arterial umbilical line
• To give an exchange blood transfusion.

When the immediate emergency's over, the doctor will probably replace the venous umbilical line with a peripheral I.V. line or an arterial umbilical line.

An arterial line is used primarily to monitor blood gas measurements, acid base status, and blood pressure. When the infant no longer needs frequent monitoring but still needs fluids, the arterial umbilical line's replaced by a peripheral I.V. line.

As useful as an umbilical line is, it carries significant risks, among them renal damage, infection, vascular perforation, hemorrhage, and damage to an extremity from arterial occlusion or spasm. As a rule, an umbilical line's not used if there's an acceptable alternative.

Your role: During and after an umbilical catheter insertion

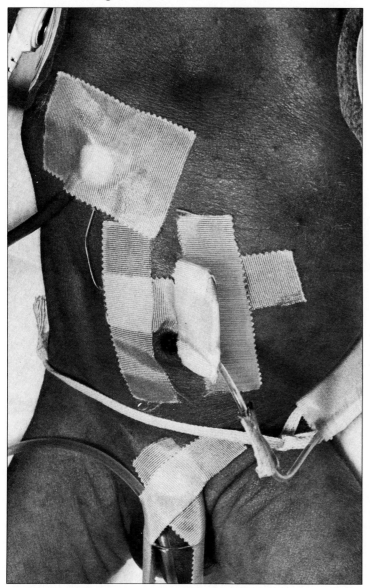

Suppose you're helping the doctor while he inserts an umbilical catheter. Whether he's establishing an arterial line or a venous line, your responsibilities are the same. In addition to gathering the equipment, you should:
• Make sure a consent form's been signed by one of the infant's parents, if your hospital requires one for this procedure.
• Make sure the infant's under a radiant heater or on a heating blanket throughout the procedure, particularly if he's premature.
• During the procedure, continually monitor the infant's vital signs and neurologic status. Be alert for any signs of distress. For example, if he develops an arterial spasm or occlusion when an arterial catheter's inserted, it may cause the leg on that side of his body to blanch. Tell the doctor at once. He'll have to withdraw the catheter and use the other artery.
• After the insertion, get an X-ray to confirm proper placement. Why? Because an incorrectly placed catheter can cause serious complications. For example, in a venous insertion, a catheter lodged in the portal venous system may cause portal vein thrombosis or spontaneous perforation of the colon. And if a hypertonic solution's fed into the portal system, liver necrosis may result.
• After the doctor's sutured and taped the catheter in place, check the markings on the side of the catheter to determine how much has been inserted. Document it. Periodically, check the catheter's length and notify the doctor immediately if any change occurs.

When the procedure's completed, your role becomes even more important. First, you must position the infant in the Isolette in a way that he can't disturb the catheter, tubing, or stopcock when he moves. Any disconnection in the line could lead to a serious, possibly fatal, hemorrhage.

Watch the infant closely for complications, which may develop rapidly and unexpectedly. Stay alert for even subtle changes in his condition: for example, irritability, lethargy, pallor, and changes in bowel movements or respiratory rate. Remember, as a nursery nurse, you'll probably be the first to notice anything unusual.

Periodically, the doctor will want lab studies done on the infant's blood. Withdraw the minimum amount necessary for each sample, and document *exactly how much blood was withdrawn* in your nurses' notes. Remember, if you must withdraw 10% to 15% of the infant's total blood volume for a sample, the doctor may want to replace it with a blood transfusion.

Any time you withdraw a blood sample or give medication, flush the catheter with heparin solution afterward. Then, include the amount of heparin solution you've injected into the line when you document the infant's daily fluid and electrolyte intake.

Delivery room crisis: Don't forget the mother

At first, the delivery of Margaret Belen's daughter seems perfectly normal. But right after birth, the infant suddenly begins gasping for air. A quick examination reveals a weak pulse, irregular heartbeat, and rapidly falling blood pressure.

The doctor acts quickly. After putting the infant under a radiant heater and giving her oxygen, he inserts a venous catheter into the umbilical cord and immediately begins a bolus infusion of I.V. sodium bicarbonate, epinephrine, and glucose. Then, he gives you the O.K. to take the infant to the neonatal ICU.

In all the excitement, you've almost forgotten about Mrs. Belen, who's watched the unexpected flurry of activity with horror. "What's wrong with my baby?" she asks you apprehensively. What should you say?

First, don't brush off her question with well-intentioned but false reassurances. If she's alert enough to know something's wrong, she won't be satisfied with a cheery, "Don't worry. Everything's fine." Instead, explain the problem in simple, direct words, avoiding clinical terms like NICU that she might not understand. For example, tell her that her baby's having difficulty breathing, and the nurses are taking her to a special nursery for care. Assure her that she'll see her baby later.

Suppose you're not sure *what's* wrong. Be honest about it, but explain what's being done to find out. Then, tell her the doctor will give her more details later, and follow up to make sure he does. Above all, remember that the stress of the delivery has reduced her ability to cope. Provide gentle, compassionate support.

Umbilical lines

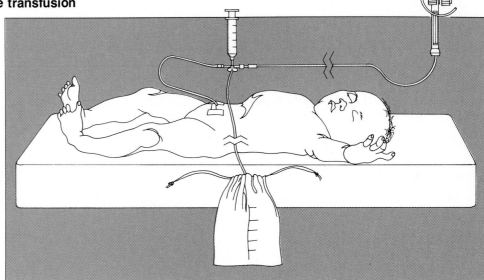

Helping the doctor perform an exchange transfusion

Suppose you're assisting with the delivery of Mrs. Crawford's third child. The doctor's told you that her second child developed erythroblastosis fetalis soon after birth. Should you expect complications with this infant too?

Yes. Chances are, Mrs. Crawford's third child also will suffer from erythroblastosis fetalis. If the infant's condition becomes acute, the doctor will treat it by performing an exchange transfusion through the infant's umbilical vein. To help him assess the infant's condition, he'll draw blood samples from the umbilical vein and send them to the lab for analysis. *Important:* To make catheter insertion easier, the doctor will leave the umbilical cord 1" to 1½" long. He'll expect you to wrap it in saline-soaked gauze to keep it from drying out.

If the doctor decides to perform an exchange transfusion, he'll want you and another nurse to help in the following ways:
• by monitoring the infant's vital signs throughout the procedure
• by recording the volume of blood withdrawn and injected, and by carefully preparing and labeling all blood samples for the lab.

Always stay alert for complications. Tell the doctor immediately if you notice *any change* in the infant's heart rate, respirations, reflexes, or temperature.

Now, let's discuss the procedure. First, the doctor will insert the correct-sized catheter into the infant's umbilical vein and attach a three-way stopcock to the catheter. Next, he'll withdraw 5 to 20 ml of blood and discard it. (By creating a slight deficit in the infant's blood volume, he guards against creating a fluid overload during the transfusion.) Then, he'll withdraw another 5 to 20 ml of the infant's blood and inject an equal amount of properly typed and cross-matched *donor* blood. He'll repeat this

exchange process until he's replaced most of the infant's blood with donor blood.

How does the doctor know how much blood to exchange? First, he calculates the infant's blood volume by estimating 85 ml of blood for each kilogram of body weight. Then, he doubles that figure to determine the amount of blood to exchange. For example, if the infant weighs 2 kg, he calculates the infant's blood volume to be 170 ml. Then, he doubles the volume and exchanges 340 ml of blood. This procedure, called a double-volume exchange, replaces 95% to 97% of the infant's original blood volume.

Since any massive blood transfusion can cause a calcium deficiency, the doctor will also inject calcium into the infant's umbilical vein during the procedure. As you probably know, calcium can slow the heart rate if injected too rapidly. So, monitor the infant's apical heart rate carefully throughout the procedure. If it falls below 80

beats per minute, tell the doctor immediately. (Of course, if the heart rate rises above 170 beats per minute, tell the doctor that too.)

When the procedure's completed, expect the doctor to draw another blood sample for lab analysis. Make sure it's labeled correctly and immediately sent to the lab. Then document the entire procedure—including the exact amounts of blood withdrawn and injected—in your nurses' notes.

Note: Suppose an infant's born with neonatal polycythemia (thick blood syndrome). This condition, if left untreated, can lead to congestive heart failure, pulmonary edema, stroke, or cardiomegaly. To correct it, the doctor will probably do a *partial* blood exchange transfusion through the infant's umbilical cord vein. During the procedure, he'll remove some of the infant's blood—thus reducing surplus of red blood cells—and replace it with a precalculated amount of fresh frozen plasma.

Why an infant may need an exchange blood transfusion

An infant suffering from erythroblastosis fetalis may need an exchange blood transfusion within several days after birth. But do you know why? Here's a brief explanation.

Erythroblastosis fetalis is usually caused by an Rh or ABO incompatibility between mother and child. The blood incompatibility triggers antibody production in the mother's blood. These antibodies attack the infant's red blood cells, causing them to hemolyze.

One result of hemolysis is the release of

excess bilirubin in the infant's bloodstream, called hyperbilirubinemia. (Although neonatal hyperbilirubinemia is usually caused by a blood incompatibility, it also may be caused by other disorders; like hepatic immaturity or biliary duct atresia.)

As the infant's bilirubin level rises, he becomes noticeably jaundiced. If his bilirubin level becomes high enough to cause kernicterus, the infant may suffer permanent brain damage. An exchange transfusion prevents this by removing excess bilirubin

from his bloodstream.

If the infant's bilirubin level isn't *dangerously* high, the doctor will probably try to control it with phototherapy first. If that doesn't help, he'll perform an exchange transfusion. *Note:* Phototherapy only affects the bilirubin level; it doesn't stop hemolysis. That's why the infant may develop severe anemia even if his bilirubin level is under control. If he does, he'll need an exchange transfusion to replace his hemolyzed red blood cells with healthy ones.

Selected references

Books

AMA DRUG EVALUATIONS, 3rd ed. Littleton, Mass.: Publishing Sciences Group, Inc., 1977.

ASSESSING VITAL FUNCTIONS ACCURATELY. Nursing Skillbook® Series. Springhouse, Pa.: Intermed Communications, Inc., 1977.

BLOOD COMPONENT THERAPY: A PHYSICIAN'S HANDBOOK. Washington, D.C.: American Association of Blood Banks, 1975.

Brunner and Suddarth. LIPPINCOTT MANUAL OF NURSING PRACTICE. Philadelphia: J.B. Lippincott Co., 1978.

Fischer, Josef. TOTAL PARENTERAL NUTRITION. Boston: Little, Brown & Co., 1976.

GENERAL PRINCIPLES OF BLOOD TRANSFUSION. Chicago: American Medical Association, 1970.

Greendyke, Robert M., and Jane C. Banzhaf. INTRODUCTION TO BLOOD BANKING, 2nd ed. Garden City, N.Y.: Medical Examination Publishing Company, 1974.

A GUIDE TO I.V. ADMIXTURE COMPATIBILITY, rev. ed. Albany, N.Y.: Delmar Publishers, 1977.

Holland, Jeanne. CARDIOVASCULAR NURSING. Boston: Little, Brown & Co., 1977.

Hudak, Carolyn M., Thelma Lohr, et al. CRITICAL CARE NURSING, 2nd ed. New York: J.B. Lippincott Co., 1977.

Mollison, P.L. BLOOD TRANSFUSION IN CLINICAL MEDICINE, 5th ed. New York: J.B. Lippincott Co. (Blackwell Scientific), 1972.

MONITORING FLUIDS AND ELECTROLYTES PRECISELY. Nursing Skillbook® Series. Springhouse, Pa.: Intermed Communications, Inc., 1978.

NEEDLE AND CANNULA TECHNIQUES. North Chicago: Abbott Laboratories, 1971.

PARENTERAL ADMINISTRATION. North Chicago: Abbott Laboratories, 1959.

Phillips, I., et al. MICROBIOLOGICAL HAZARDS OF INFUSION THERAPY. Littleton, Mass.: Publishing Sciences Group, Inc., 1976.

Plumer, Ada L. PRINCIPLES AND PRACTICES OF INTRAVENOUS THERAPY, 2nd ed. Boston: Little, Brown & Co., 1975.

STANDARDS FOR BLOOD BANKS AND TRANSFUSION SERVICES, 9th ed. Washington, D.C.: American Association of Blood Banks, 1978.

Storlie, Frances. PATIENT TEACHING IN CRITICAL CARE. New York: Appleton-Century-Crofts, 1975.

Trissel, Lawrence. PARENTERAL DRUG INFORMATION GUIDE. Washington, D.C.: American Society of Hospital Pharmacists, 1974.

Worley, Eloise. PHARMACOLOGY AND MEDICATIONS, 3rd ed. Philadelphia: F.A. Davis Co., 1976.

Periodicals

Adams, Nancy. *Reducing the Perils of Intracardiac Monitoring,* NURSING76. 6:66-74, April 1976.

Beaumont, Estelle. *The New I.V. Infusion Pumps,* NURSING77. 7:31-35, July 1977.

Haughey, B. *CVP Lines: Monitoring and Maintaining,* AMERICAN JOURNAL OF NURSING. 78:635-638, April 1978.

Tinker, J. *Two Methods of Assessing the Critically Ill Patient,* Part 2, NURSING TIMES. 74:318-320, February 23, 1978.

Acknowledgements

We'd like to thank the following people and companies for their help with this PHOTOBOOK:

ABBOTT LABORATORIES
North Chicago, Ill.
Barry Wawrzyn,
Marketing Manager
Joan Spece Worley
Steven Ulrich

AMERICAN RED CROSS
Philadelphia, Pa.

AUTO-SYRINGE, INC.
Hooksett, N.H.
Bill Arthur,
Vice President Marketing & Sales

BARD-PARKER
Division Becton Dickinson and Company
Lincoln Park, N.J.
Edward F. Lanoue,
Product Manager

CONCORD LABORATORIES, INC.
Keane, N.H.
Michael Weldon,
Advertising Manager

FENWAL LABORATORIES
Division of Travenol Laboratories, Inc.
Deerfield, Ill.
Ronald F. Frantz,
Marketing Communications Manager
Jim Gosnay

HEALTHCO, INC.
Reading, Pa.
Al Szymborski, CMR

IVAC CORPORATION
San Diego, Calif.
Chérie M. Hawes, RN,
Clinical Specialist

JELCO LABORATORIES
Raritan, N.J.
Candace Neale-May,
Product Manager

McGAW LABORATORIES
Newport Beach, Calif.
Val Montegrande,
Marketing Communications Manager

MERCK SHARP & DOHME
West Point, Pa.

SORENSON RESEARCH COMPANY
Trevose, Pa.
R. James Jones,
Eastern Zone Manager

TRAVENOL LABORATORIES, INC.
Deerfield, Ill.

Also the staffs of:

ALBERT EINSTEIN MEDICAL CENTER
Northern Division
Philadelphia, Pa.

DELAWARE VALLEY MEDICAL CENTER
Bristol, Pa.

JEANES HOSPITAL
Philadelphia, Pa.

TEMPLE UNIVERSITY HOSPITAL
Philadelphia, Pa.

Patient teaching aid

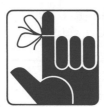

Preparing the pediatric patient for I.V. therapy

Does giving I.V. therapy to a child present special problems for you? Perhaps this teaching aid will help. The drawings to the right are a miniature version of the coloring booklet which follows. We suggest that you photocopy several sets of the next 4 pages. Then, when you must give an I.V. to a pediatric patient, bring one of these coloring booklets and some crayons or colored pencils to your patient teaching session.

Sit down and talk things over. If your patient is under age 7, read the booklet to him. Give him plenty of time to ask questions and answer honestly. Then suggest he color in the pages of the booklet as he likes.

If your patient is over age 7, encourage him to read the booklet himself. But be sure to allow plenty of time to answer any questions he may have. A child over age 7 may also want to color the pictures, but he may prefer using colored pencils.

Nursing tip: Show your continued interest in your patient by asking him to show you the booklet when he's finished coloring the pictures. Also encourage him to show it to his parents, his doctor, and his other visitors.

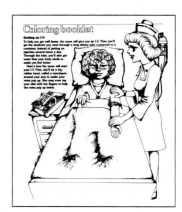
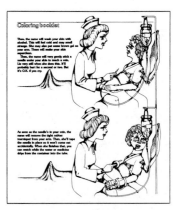
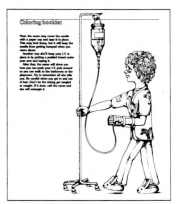
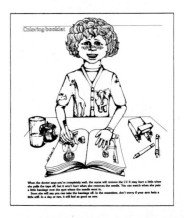

Coloring booklet

Getting an I.V.

To help you get well faster, the nurse will give you an I.V. Then you'll get the medicine you need through a long skinny tube connected to a container, instead of getting an injection several times a day. Through the tube, you'll also get water that your body needs to make you feel better.

Here's how the nurse will start your I.V. First, she'll tie a big rubber band, called a tourniquet, around your arm to make your veins pop up. She may even tap your skin with her fingers to help the veins pop up better.

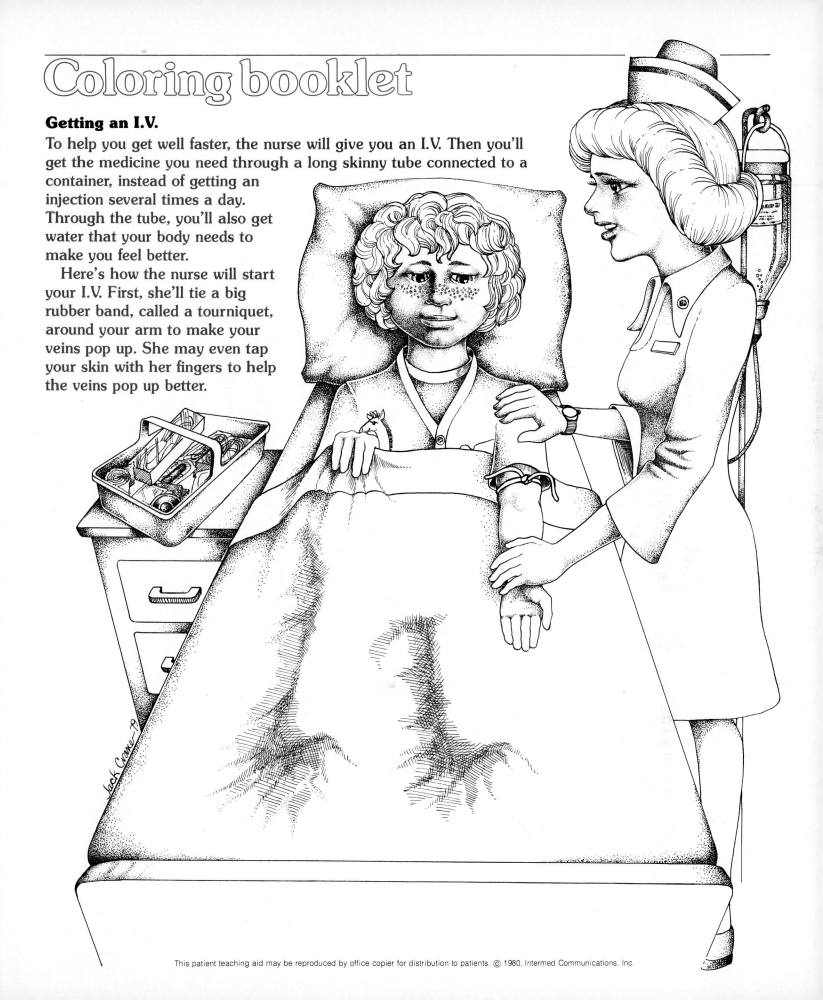

This patient teaching aid may be reproduced by office copier for distribution to patients. © 1980, Intermed Communications, Inc.

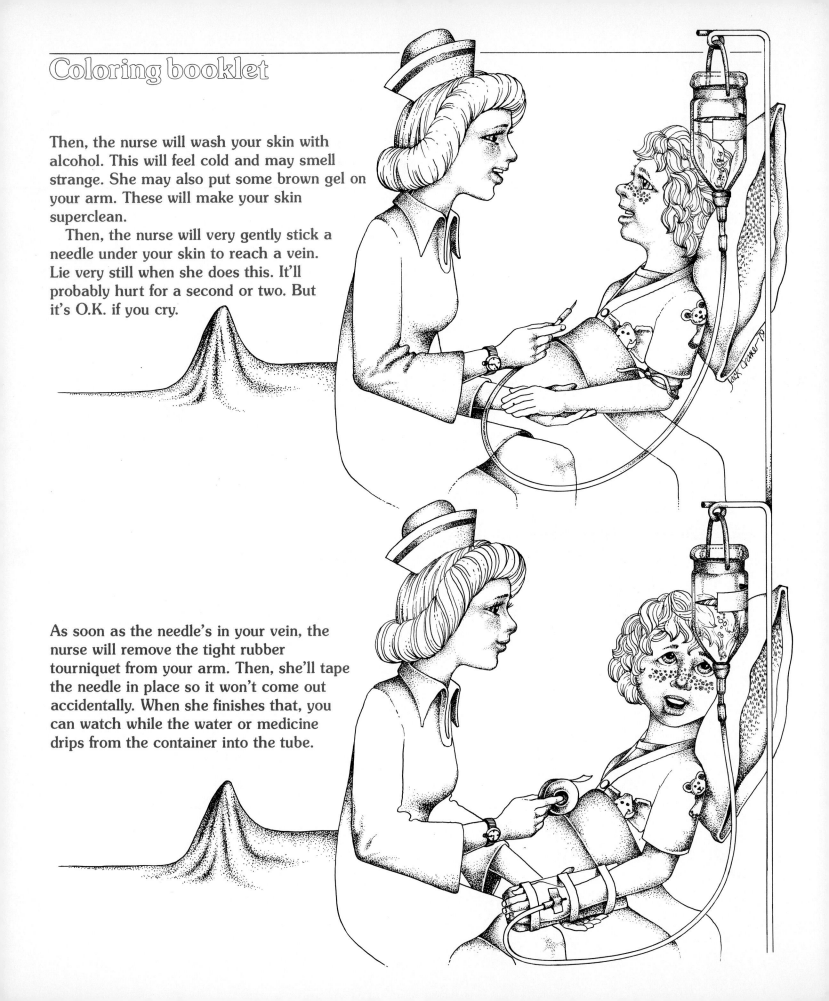

Then, the nurse will wash your skin with alcohol. This will feel cold and may smell strange. She may also put some brown gel on your arm. These will make your skin superclean.

Then, the nurse will very gently stick a needle under your skin to reach a vein. Lie very still when she does this. It'll probably hurt for a second or two. But it's O.K. if you cry.

As soon as the needle's in your vein, the nurse will remove the tight rubber tourniquet from your arm. Then, she'll tape the needle in place so it won't come out accidentally. When she finishes that, you can watch while the water or medicine drips from the container into the tube.

Next, the nurse may cover the needle with a paper cup and tape it in place. This may look funny, but it will keep the needle from getting bumped when you move about.

Another way she'll keep your I.V. in place is by putting a padded board under your arm and taping it.

After that, the nurse will show you how you can push your I.V. pole around so you can walk to the bathroom or the playroom. Try to remember all she tells you. Be careful when you get in and out of bed. Don't let the tubing get tangled or caught. If it does, call the nurse and she will untangle it.

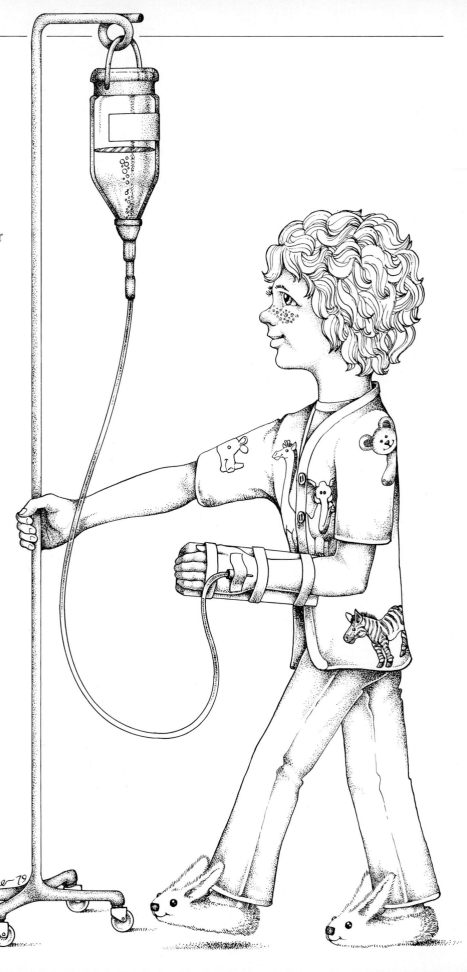

Jack Crane—79

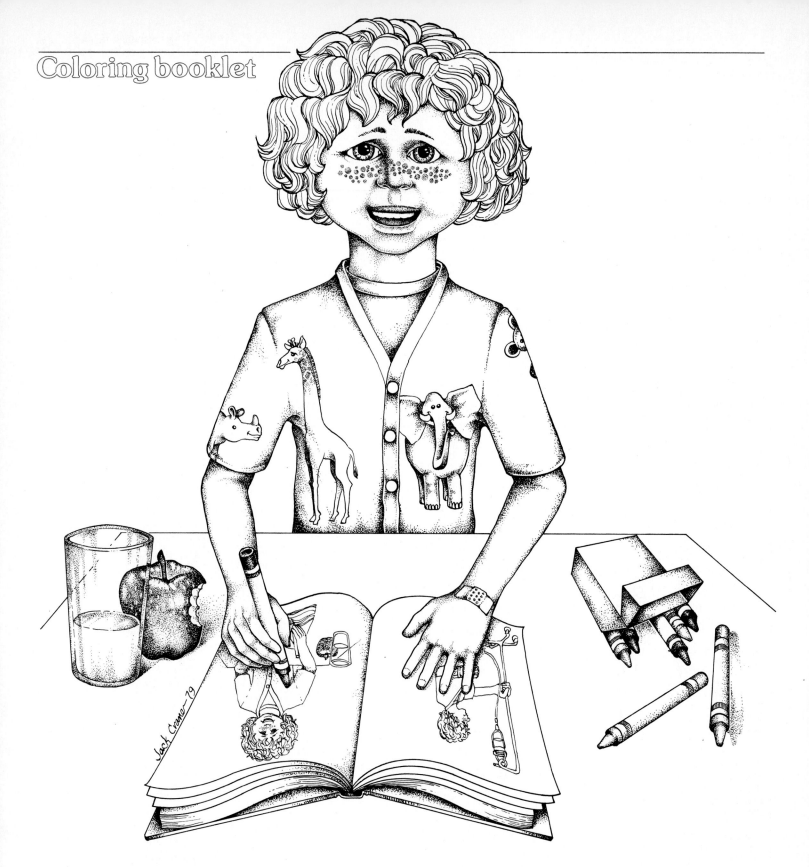

When the doctor says you're completely well, the nurse will remove the I.V. It may hurt a little when she pulls the tape off, but it won't hurt when she removes the needle. You can watch when she puts a little bandage over the spot where the needle went in.

Soon she will say you can take the bandage off. In the meantime, don't worry if your arm feels a little stiff. In a day or two, it will feel as good as new.

Index

A

Abbott Accuprime adapter, 54-55
Abbott/Shaw LifeCare Pump®.
See *I.V. pumps and controllers, piston pump.*
Accuprime adapter. See *Abbott Accuprime adapter.*
Add-a-filter. See *Needle filters.*
Additive cap, 13, 66
Additive sets, 71-80. See also *Volume-control sets.*
  equipment, 72
  indications/contraindications, 72
  patient preparation, 72
  problems, 76, 80
  setting up a partial-fill piggyback set, 74-75
  setting up a secondary set, 73
Admixtures. See *I.V. admixtures.*
Air embolism, 58, 100-101, 124
Albumin, 114-115
Allergic reaction
  blood, 124
  I.V. therapy, 59
Ambulatory patient, 60
Ampule transfer device, 69
Antecubital fossa. See also *Venipuncture, site selection.*
  anatomy, 27
  description of, 28
Artery
  anatomy, 26-27, 28
  umbilical, 148-149
Aseptic technique, 11
Automatic infiltration detector (Abbott/Shaw LifeCare Pump), 56
Auto-Syringe Syringe Pump. See *I.V. pumps and controllers, syringe pump.*

B

Backcheck valve. See *Ports, piggyback.*
Backflow. See *Blood backflow.*
Bedridden patient, 60
Bevel positioning. See *Needles and cannulas, bevel positioning.*
Blood ammonia level, 132
Blood backflow, 34
Blood contamination, 124
Blood donation, 125
Blood pump
  built-in, 126-127
  slip-on, 128-129
Blood requisition form, 113
Blood transfusions, 112-134
  blood-warming coil, 130
  built-in blood pump, 126-127
  complications
    equipment, 125
    immediate reactions, 124

massive transfusions, 132
transmittal diseases, 133
component drip set, 123
component syringe set, 122-123
documenting, 134
electric blood warmer, 131
exchange, 148, 150
hazards, 113
indications/contraindications, 114-115
introduction to, 112
microaggregate recipient set, 118-119
patient care, 125
requisition forms, 113
Rh factor, 113
slip-on blood pump, 128-129
special considerations, 115
straight-line blood set, 116-117
typing and crossmatching, 113, 115
Y-set, 120-121
Blood warmer, electric, 131
Blood-warming coil, 130
Buffers, 64
Buretrol® See *Volume-control sets.*
Butterfly needle. See *Winged-tip needle.*

C

Cannula, 18. See also *INC, ONC.*
Carbohydrates in sodium chloride solution, 12
Carbohydrates in water, 12
Catheter embolism, 42, 59, 105
Central line, direct, 92
  changing dressing, 102-103
  changing tubing, 101
  complications, 100-101, 103
  confirming proper placement, 97
  CVP insertion, 140
  insertion, 94-97
  maintaining, 97
  removal, 104-105
  site anatomy, 26
  taping and dressing, 96-97
Central line, jugular, 92
  complications, 100-101, 103
  insertion, 99
  site anatomy, 26
Central line, peripheral, 92
  complications, 98, 100-101, 103
  insertion, 98
  site anatomy, 27
Central venous pressure, 140-145. See also *Central line, direct.*
  interpreting reading, 145

one-piece manometer, 145
patient care, 145
setting up CVP manometer, 141-142
taking reading, 142-145
Charting. See *Documenting.*
Chevron method. See *Taping and dressing, chevron method.*
Children's coloring booklet, 152
Circulatory overload, 58
  in blood transfusion, 124, 136
Clamps. See *Flow clamps.*
CMV virus, 133
Compatibility and stability
  of I.V. admixtures, 64
  of I.V. bolus, 86
Component drip set, 123
Component syringe set, 122-123
Controllers. See *I.V. pumps and controllers.*
Crankcase spool catheter, 98
Crossmatching, blood, 113
Cryoprecipitate concentrate administration, 122-123
Cutdown, 19, 146-147
  equipment, 146
  performing a, 146-147
  removing catheter, 147
  site selection, 146
CVP manometer, 141-145
  one-piece, 145
  setting up, 141-142
  taking reading, 142-145

D

Dextrose and saline solution. See *Carbohydrates in sodium chloride solution.*
Dextrose and water. See *Carbohydrates in water.*
Dilating a vein. See *Vein, dilation.*
Direct central line. See *Central line, direct.*
Direct method of insertion, 35
Documenting
  basic I.V. therapy, 43
  blood requisition form, 113
  blood transfusion, 134
  central line removal, 105
  phlebotomy, 136
Dorsum of the hand
  anatomy, 27
Double-headed pin, 68
Dressings. See also *Taping and dressing.*
  changing, basic I.V., 47
  hyperalimentation and, 96-97, 102-103
  jugular vein line and, 92
Drip systems, 14. See also *Macrodrip and Microdrip.*
  flow rate calculation, 17

Index

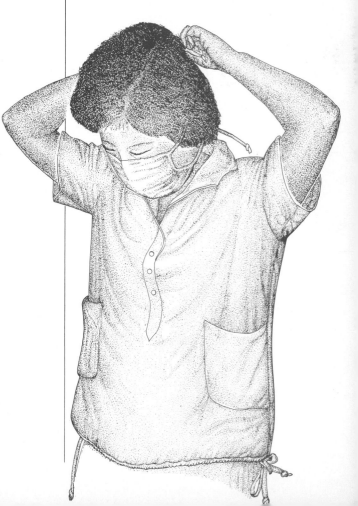

Index

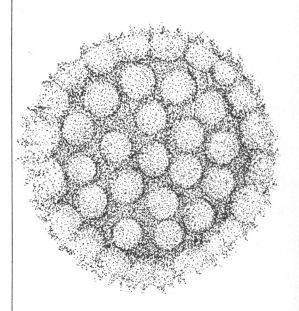